I HAD KILLER BOOBS

How I Slayed My Tumor
with Sass & Humor

by LUCY BEATO

All Rights Reserved

COPYRIGHT © 2022 Lucy Beato

This book may not be reproduced, transmitted, or stored in whole or in part by any means, including graphic, electronic, or mechanical, without the express written consent of the publisher except in the case of brief questions embodied in critical articles and reviews.

ISBN: 979-8-218-02644-8

Table of Contents

Acknowledgments i
Preface iii
Introduction 1
Chapter 1 – Plot Twist (Cancer) 3
Chapter 2 – It's Official… I Have Killer Boobs! 11
Chapter 3 – My Boobs, First in Line 19
Chapter 4 – Goodbye, Boobies 25
Chapter 5 – One Cancer for All 33
Chapter 6 – Thanks for the Mamories 41
Chapter 7 – Can You Add Some Tequila to That Cocktail? 49
Chapter 8 – A Boss Lady Fighting Cancer 63
Chapter 9 – Fighting Chemons and My Multiple Personalities ... 69
Chapter 10 – Cancer Survival Kit 77
Chapter 11 – I Don't Mean to Brag But… I Just Beat Cancer 85
Chapter 12 – Until Cancer Do Us Part 91
Chapter 13 – A Little Stitious 97
Chapter 14 – Well, That Didn't Go As Planned! 99
Chapter 15 – Wait, One More Thing… 105
Final Message 109
About the Author 112

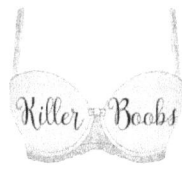

Acknowledgments

> *"Feeling gratitude and not expressing it is like wrapping a present and not giving it."*
> —William Arthur Ward

No one who beats cancer does it without acknowledging the support of others. I would like to recognize and give my warmest thanks to a few special people for making my voyage to *Cancerville* much more pleasant and smooth.

First and foremost, to God for believing I was a lean, mean, cancer-fighting machine. Thank you, God, for the trust. I know you had a plan, and that is always perfect. However, I want to let you know that I learned my lesson and I'm strong enough already, thanks! Also, thank you for giving me the wisdom to transform my tragedy into comedy. I know there is nothing funny about having cancer, but I have a great sense of tumor.

To my beloved Killer Boobs, who I miss, but who have inspired and given me something to talk about. Without their support, this book would have never been written.

To my warrior mom, whose faith and resilience are admirable. Mom, I know you have earned special privileges with the one from above. I am 100 % confident that your prayers saved my life.

To my sister, my keeper, for your help, comfort, and most importantly, for making me realize that one can never trust a lump.

To my adorable children for giving me superpowers and the courage to become a Cool Mom fighting cancer.

To all of Team Lucy, for being like my perfect bra, supportive, and for never leaving me hanging.

To my amazing team of doctors who saved my life and had to put up with my interrogations and my paranoia.

To all the special people in my life who kept me going, encouraged me, and cheered me to make this book possible.

And last but not least, to you, my wonderful readers, for allowing me to share my boob tale.

Thank you all from the bottom of my heart.

Cancer… Been there, Beat that.

—Lucy

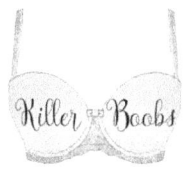

Preface

Warning:

If you picked up this book to read, it's likely for one of the following reasons:

1. You are battling cancer and need some inspiration and humor. If that's the case, congratulations, you are a champ, and you've got this. Keep going, don't let cancer distract you.

2. You know someone who is battling cancer and want to recommend her this book. If that's the case, please pick up two extra copies and pay it forward.

3. You are a relative or a friend who wants to support me or is just curious about my journey or writing. If that is the case, stop at this very moment and check your boobs—mine tried to kill me.

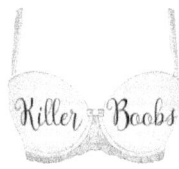

Introduction

Oh yes, my boobs are fake; my real ones tried to kill me!

Have you ever heard the term *Killer Boobs*? I promise I didn't make it up, but I did have a pair. Moreover, have you ever thought about doing something as bizarre as throwing a party for your boobs even though they wanted to kill you? Well, I did! You might think I'm crazy, and you may be right! Being diagnosed with breast cancer is not necessarily a reason to celebrate; yet I could not allow such an important milestone in my life as losing my *breasties* to go unnoticed. Perhaps they were a little asymmetrical and not the most perfect pair, but they were my pair. They fed my two babies, made my husband happy, and accentuated my feminine Latina curves. So yes, they deserved a proper farewell.

Before I share any further, let me get some things off my chest. As soon as I hit puberty, my breasts developed faster than a Polaroid. I know boobies are just fatty tissue that makes us look sexy, but mine had a little extra fat.

For many years I was a little self-conscious about my boobs because I thought they were a little too big. While Cinderella dreamed of meeting her Prince Charming, I dreamed of having smaller, perky boobs. Hey, we are all entitled to dream, and that was mine. In all honesty, they were not that big—just a small, tenacious D. Many women would pay big bucks to have that size, but not me; I was not pleased with the size and shape.

My dissatisfaction got worse after breastfeeding my two kids and gaining and losing weight. At that point, the D stood for "Deflated." Oh yes!!! My breasts were sagging and deflated. Two words that women don't necessarily want to combine in a phrase when describing their boobs. Well, that was my reality I had to live with unless I would "Marie Kondo" them, which I had no plans to do. Good thing for push-up bras; they certainly did wonders for my classy cleavage. While some women might have been envious of my curves, all I wished was not to need to hold my boobs while running down the stairs. That was challenging!

**Be careful how you treat your boobs,
they sure have a funny way of getting back at you.**

I knew sooner or later my boobs would rebel, and they sure did by surprising me with a little tumor humor. How funny was that? Well, as much as I enjoy laughing, I didn't find it funny. My boobs had betrayed me! Ironically, just when I realized that all I needed was a good pair of push-up bras. Besides, big boobs are always in style. The betrayal left me in a complete state of shock. I did not see that coming. Was this Karma? Was this a result of me constantly complaining about them? Is that why they were always sad, looking down, lifeless, and droopy? These were all the thoughts that came to mind. I felt so guilty. For so long, I was not accepting of them. In fact, all I wanted was two things: world peace and a pair of perky smaller boobs. Hmm, be careful what you wish for!

Sure enough I was about to get an involuntary boob job, a pair of new perky silicone boobs courtesy of breast cancer. Wait! Did that mean that world peace was next? I hope so because I was about to endure a war, a true cancer battle.

Going through cancer is terrifying; you experience an emotional imbalance: worry, fear, grief, uncertainty, and even anger. Despite all these feelings, I turned to humor as my coping mechanism and my best form of therapy. It helped me diminish some of those emotions and kept me sane in the midst of chaos. So, after accepting that I had killer boobs, I decided to slay my tumor with a bit of sass and humor.

Ok, I'm glad I got all that excess baggage off my chest; it was heavy. Now, let's move on!

I know there is nothing funny about cancer unless you have a sense of *tumor*, but it can certainly help you heal. Your primary focus is to beat it, but while doing so, laugh with it. Otherwise, it will kill you. Once you overcome cancer, you become sassy, unstoppable, and fearless. You are ready to act on any crazy idea that pops into your head, such as writing a book, and not just any book, a witty, heartfelt, and inspiring book that will keep you entertained, give you hope, and teach you some *blessons**. I not only share my bumpy, lumpy, and spunky ride to Cancerville, but I also share quotes, sayings, and several anecdotes that made me laugh and inspired me to put my *breast* foot forward when my motivation lapsed so I could get back on track and to finish like a boss.

Narrating my story also gave me an outlet to heal. I knew that one day I would turn my pain into purpose to serve as a source of inspiration, support, and hope for other women going through similar, life-altering experiences, and here I am! Because every survivor has stories to tell, jokes to make, and *blessons* to share, here are mine, and as I share them, I hope I can help you find your own. In the meantime, buckle up. It's about to get really lumpy.

Blesson = Blessing + Lesson- —viewing a painful lesson as a blessing.

"Life is lumpy. And a lump in the oatmeal, a lump in the throat and a lump in the breast are not the same lump. One should learn the difference."
—*Robert Fulghum*

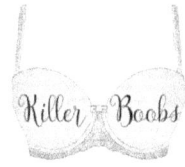

Chapter 1
Plot Twist (Cancer)

When something goes wrong in your life,
just yell 'Plot Twist' and move on.
—*Unknown*

At 39, my life was perfect. I had everything I needed to be happy and grateful—my husband, two healthy children, a dog, and a thriving business. What else could I ask for? OK, maybe it was a bit monotonous and dull, but it was my happy place. I was habitually following a strict routine that helped me balance my professional and family life, giving myself no room for something as silly as cancer. Having a routine gave me exactly what I needed—complete control. I'll admit that perhaps I was a bit of a control freak or a control enthusiast, as I would like to call it. I was completely flexible as long as everything was exactly the way I wanted. My life wasn't free of challenges, but I would buckle up and face whatever it threw at me head-on. However, sometimes a break from your routine is all that's needed to turn your life upside down and lose complete control over it.

It was a typical Thursday. After work, I did all my daily duties: cooking, cleaning, homework, planning, playing, etc.—you know, the usual for us moms. Then, I headed to the gym. Call me crazy but somehow exhausting myself at the gym was the most relaxing part of my day. I came home filled with energy and headed into the shower to relax before I could enjoy a good night's sleep. I cannot even begin to tell how much I love standing under the warm water, letting it hit my sore muscles and untying the exhaustion knots in my body. In addition to making you sound like a great singer, taking a shower also helps you contemplate life's most challenging decisions. Little did I know I was about to have to make some tough ones as that shower turned out to be life-altering, or should I say life-saving?

Suddenly the urge to do a "self-exam" sprung up in my heart. You know that little voice in your head that says, "*Touch your boobs,*" and you follow her advice, not knowing exactly why. Then, boom!!

I Felt a Lump...

Gee, what is that? Is it all in my head? It doesn't hurt, so I'm good. Quickly brushing away the thought of anything being out of the norm, I took a flight back to reality, where everything was perfect for me. Having a tumor? Nah, ain't nobody got time for that. Days passed, and without a care in the world, I followed my routine like a pro. The thought of the lump would pop up sporadically. I had a feeling something was a little off with me. I mean, I'm not that normal as it is, but something was up. Maybe it was stress from being a super mom, super wife, super boss, and super tired. Who knows, but I had not been myself for a few weeks. I hate being suspicious, but damn, that gut feeling hardly ever fails.

Feeling for lumps can save your bumps.

I decided to monitor my breast daily. Are you there? Yup, still here!!! OK, I'll check again tomorrow. At first, it only had my curiosity, but now it had my attention. More so because my body was sending me signals (e.g., headaches, lack of focus, feeling low, and sadness seeping in). I'm sure it was nothing related to my tumor, but the signs worried me.

I decided to get a second opinion, not from a doctor, but from my husband. Who would know the *size* and *shape* of it better than him? Why didn't it occur to me before? I asked him, "Can you please touch my breast?" He looked at me as if I were crazy because I'm usually not that blunt. "I think I have a lump." I exclaimed. After feeling it, his answer did not surprise me. "Yes," he affirmed. "*I could tell even from a distance,*" he added. Determined not to allow his dramatic answer to worry me, I laughed at his comment, given that he always liked to embellish the facts.

The doubt had already crept in, so I decided to tell my sister because she is my go-to person in times of doubt. I called her, expecting to hear a comforting reaction from her, such as, "*Oh, no worries. It's probably just a lump of fat.*" Instead, she immediately suggested that I make an appointment to see the doctor. Oh gosh, let's call my sister "Dramatic Debbie." I should have kept my mouth shut. *Was she my big sister or little sister? Was she the boss of me who thinks she can tell me what to do?* I thought in disbelief. She was not kidding and kept insisting until I finally made an appointment to see the doctor, even though I was sure it was *"just a lump of fat"* that would be gone in no time.

Cancer... No, Not Me!

While driving to the doctor, I was surrounded by all forms of doubts. On the one hand, I was sure such things did not happen to young and healthy women. On the other hand, my anxiety was rising as I feared the "lump of fat" in my body could actually be a tumor.

Surprisingly, the appointment went well, and the doctor assured me it was probably fatty tissue. *"Oh, thank God,"* I thought to myself. As suspected, just an indolent lump of fat. She did order a mammogram and a sonogram to rule out any doubts. At this moment, the rushing relief that I felt was similar to what a mother feels when her baby finally falls asleep at 3 am. Doctors are the experts, aren't they? So, I had nothing to worry about. I was convinced that my sister was being *"Dramatic Debbie,"* and I couldn't wait to tell her it was just a bad joke.

Just a Pinch on My Boob

At my follow-up visit to review the results, the doctor confirmed that there was a lump and ordered a biopsy, which triggered my deepest fears. Things were getting serious. A BIOPSY! "Oh yes, I love needles. Let's get a biopsy," said no one ever. I wondered, "Why in the world am I being asked to get a biopsy for just 'a lump of fat'? Didn't the doctor confirm that everything was OK?" Then, I thought, "It's just a pinch on my boob. Let's just get it over with." Nothing to stress about; it will be OK.

I was somewhat okay with it until I was hit with a $1600 deductible. Wait, what? Hold on; this whole biopsy was not even my idea! Whoever invites pays! So, I shouldn't have to pay for it. The cost made me rethink my decision. I had other priorities, you know, like a pair of red-bottomed shoes or a nice LV bag, essential accessories we women always all need. In the meantime, what over-the-counter medicine can I take for my possible life-threatening "lump of fat" to avoid paying for this? Clearly, I had my priorities, and this lump was not one. Hey, don't judge. I know I'm not the only woman who does not prioritize health at times. It happens to the best of us. I did learn my lesson.

While trying to convince myself not to get the biopsy, the little voice inside me had another point of view. It kept lingering in my head. I finally listened to it and decided to get my boob pinched. Better to be safe than sorry.

Biopsy or Autopsy, Not Sure!

It was time for the *Biopsy*. Thinking that I was Superwoman, ready to take on even the toughest of adversaries, I headed to my appointment alone. I had never had a needle pierce my boob, so I did not know what to expect. Let me tell you, it was agonizing. I will never forget the excruciating pain as the needle pricked my breast. Who came up with that concept? It was a biopsy, but it felt more like an autopsy. I was dying. My control over my emotions was slipping away, and the tears rolling down my cheeks were proof of it. I felt weak, which was an unfamiliar feeling. I also felt vulnerable, lonely, and scared. I knew things were getting serious. The ten minutes, which felt like an eternity, were finally over. I wiped my tears, grabbed my golden lasso, and kept moving. The worst was over; at least, I was trying to convince myself it was.

Congrats, You Have Cancer!

It was Monday, the day after my son's 3rd birthday celebration, and an easy day at my hair salon I was in great spirits. While enjoying my healthy lunch of lightly seasoned salmon, sweet potatoes, and broccoli, my waiting time was cut short as I got a call from the doctor. Thank God! Finally, I was going to be at peace knowing it was "just a lump of extra fat." "Do you have a few minutes to talk," the doctor asked. "Sure," I replied. "Just confirm everything is fine," I thought to myself.

"Your results are positive; you have invasive ductal carcinoma." "What? What is that?" I asked. "You have CANCER," she repeated. I wanted to say, "Oh no, thanks, you have the wrong number." But instead, the words hit me like a ton of bricks, and I stood completely silent.

I've heard many awful things, but this news had no comparison. CANCER and me in the same sentence??? That didn't even rhyme.

The doctor overwhelmed me with information, but I was mentally numb and unable to process what she said afterward. I was in complete shock.

I remained calm and composed while pretending to listen but burst into tears once I hung up the phone. The "control" I was so used to had gone down the drain. I stopped eating my lunch, gathered all my belongings, and rushed to my car. I wanted to be alone. As a business owner, being seen in such a vulnerable state was not normal for me. I had to maintain my composure, but who can in the middle of a crisis?

My Six Stages of Grief

As I sat in my car sobbing like a baby after hearing the shocking news, there was still some hope deep inside. Part of me thought, "You have nothing to worry about." They say, *"A bad weed never dies,"* but they also say, *"Good things don't last."* So, I wasn't really sure where I stood. Was I going to die or not? Over the next two hours, I experienced all the stages of grief:

1. *Denial.* This must be a mistake. I eat my veggies and an apple a day, and I exercise. Doctors misdiagnose patients all the time. Besides, I have lumps of fat all over my thighs—are those also tumors? I need a second opinion!

2. *Anger.* It is only February—what happened to my New Year's resolution that this would be my year? Why me? I'm a good woman. What did I do to deserve this? How can this be happening to me? God, if this was part of your plan, you are a terrible planner! You are being unfair!

3. *Bargaining.* Oh God, sorry! Please, let this be a mistake. I was kidding. You are fair, and your plans are always perfect. It's not you; it's me. I promise I'll stop being such a control enthusiast and will never doubt you. I will pray day and night. God, I beg you, please!

4. *Depression.* My life is over! I'm going to die. What will happen to my kids and my business? Who am I going to inspire now with an unhealthy tumor? How can I come back from this? So much for

eating broccoli and kale. Unhealthy me! I'm such a disappointment!

5. *Acceptance.* OK, fine. I have cancer, but it's not my fault. I didn't let it in. It broke in. So, yes, I have cancer, but cancer doesn't have me!!!

6. **Determination.** I can't afford to die. My family needs me, and the world needs me. I am an ass-kicking, fire-breathing, dragon beast, cancer-fighting machine, and I will handle this s#!+!

And just like that, my perfectly planned life had a plot twist.

Ugh, I just finished unloading some heavy baggage, but where is the humor? Not sure, but it needed to be confessed to clear the lumpy road. In retrospect, my entire life had been based on planning a "perfect life:" graduate from high school, go to college, get a degree, get married, become an entrepreneur, build a family, achieve holistic success, and live happily ever after.

I really wanted a perfect ending, but I had to learn the hard way that:

"Unexpected things were always going to happen in life and that the only control I had was how I was going to handle them. So, I decided to survive using courage, humor, and grace. I was the queen of my own life, and the choice was mine."

—Queenism

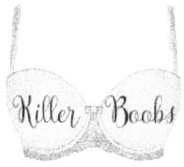

Chapter 2

It's Official... I Have Killer Boobs!

Yes, but you are a badass,
and you will fight with your superpowers.

To say that my family thought I was stronger than a rock was an understatement. They sure thought I had superpowers. Maybe it was my ability to remain calm, my determination to rise no matter how difficult the situation, or simply because I worked out and had muscles, I don't know. Still, I truly believe they thought I was Wonder Woman, which was alarming.

Something Funny Happened Today!

Picking up my kids from school that day was tough. Seeing their happy faces and knowing what I was about to put them through was heartbreaking, but I kept my composure. I had not practiced the part of the script in the book of life where I had to reveal such tragic news. So, amid my sadness, we drove home, summarizing their day and singing their favorite songs as usual.

When we got home, my husband was cooking dinner. I went straight to my room to practice how I would break the news. I should say, "*I have cancer,*" or "*Hey, guess what? I have cancer,*" or "*Something funny happened today; I have killer boobs.*" I practiced using different tones and voices a few times not to sound so dramatic before finally breaking the news.

"Food is ready," he yelled. Oh Lord, I wasn't ready to confront him, and for the first time in a long time, I wasn't hungry, something very uncommon to me, as eating is one of my favorite hobbies. He noticed I didn't come downstairs despite the announcements, and I think he sensed something was not right. So, he came upstairs. "I have cancer," I yelled as soon as he entered the room. I needed to get it off my chest immediately. Boy, my chest held a lot of things!

The room became as quiet as a baseball field during the off-season. His response was less dramatic than expected. In fact, it was as cold as ice. My husband's love was like a toothache; it doesn't show up in x-rays, but you know it's there. He stood in complete silence, and although I could tell he was shaken, he kept his composure and replied, "You will be fine. Come eat." He always gave the impression that everything would be fine even when it seemed things were falling apart, which was always comforting. I loved my husband but felt the urge to beat him up for handling it so nonchalantly and being so sure I would beat it. Why was he so confident? It was obvious that he believed I had superpowers to resolve anything, and this was no exception.

Up next was my sister; she was eagerly waiting for me to hear back from the doctor. She called me several times that day, but I evaded her, like when a teacher asks a question, and you avoid eye contact because you don't know the answer. Well, I didn't know the answer, or should I say, I had not practiced that part of the script. My silence said it all. She suspected that something was wrong, and she was right. Finally, I answered at around 9:00 pm after about five missed calls. She knew immediately and wanted to know the details, but I had no words. She comforted me and assured me that we would get through this together. I asked her to please share the news with the rest of my immediate family, as I did not have the courage to confront them, and my script was incomplete.

Speaking to my mom after she heard the news was surreal. She was as calm as a toad in the sun. She showed no signs of worry. Deep inside, I know she was hurting because no parent wants to hear that their child has a deadly disease, no matter what age. One thing you should know about my mom is that her faith is stronger than her coffee. She would not allow my cancer to intimidate her and instead reassured me that I would be fine. I was in shock, and her reaction made me think she might be a little delusional.

My dad and brother were next in line, and again, without hesitation, they reassured me that I was going to beat it and reminded me of my strength. How did they know this? Did I have cancer before and not know it? They must have thought I was Wonder Woman, but I felt more like Wounded Woman. The pressure was on, and everyone had high expectations of me as if I were a cancer-fighting machine. I had to live up to them. Yes, they were right! I'm a tough cookie, except for cancer. Other than that, I'm fine.

Let's go to Disney, Where Miracles do Happen

"Let's go to Disney," my husband said a few days after my diagnosis. He had a very strange way of coping with pain. Who thinks of going to Disney when a family member has been hit with cancer? Well, clearly, he did. Perhaps he thought I might be done adulting, and I get it because adulting is like looking both ways before crossing the street and getting hit by a plane. Or maybe he just wanted to get me out of my funk. As optimistic as I am, I was in a funk. My life was not going as planned, and that was not OK. Trying to escape from reality, I agreed to go. I love being human, but some days I wish I could be a fairy, and this was the perfect place for it. Disney is the happiest place of all and where all dreams come true. Hey, maybe I'd become a fairy. Who knows, so let's go.

Disney was magical, and we had a great weekend. The kids, as usual, had a blast, and I made the best of it. Seeing them happy made me happy. That weekend was different; I was really able to appreciate my family, focus on being present, and not deal with work. Disconnecting from work had always been hard for me as a businesswoman. I often missed important things like quality family time and had even forgotten how precious it is to be alive and live in the moment.

Maybe Life Isn't So Magical After All

Now back to the real world after the magic is gone. Explaining to my kids that I had cancer was quite a challenge. My oldest daughter was seven, and my youngest son had recently turned three. They are happy kids with a "perfect life" that was now going to be disrupted by cancer. How do I explain this without causing them stress? I had to—you can't fool kids, well, at least not my kids. They are the most observant and inquisitive kids, especially my 3-year-old. He will ask an arsenal of questions. Kids quickly pick up on vibes and conversations no matter how much you try to hide them. I certainly did not want them to wander around with uncertainty or without understanding what was happening. I managed to find a way and explain to them the meaning of cancer, the treatment, and the changes I was about to endure.

"Are you going to die?" was their first concern. "Of course not," I replied assertively—just a few procedures to make me feel better. "Are you going to lose your hair," my 3-year-old inquired surprisingly. He had seen commercials with kids at St. Jude hospital and made the connection. How clever is that? Yup, they are my kids. My son went about his day as expected, but my daughter was slightly more concerned. I could tell she was worried; she has always been a bit mature for her age. "Oh Lord, please help me stay strong for my kids," I prayed. Have you heard the saying, "Parenting is hard?" Well, this is an excellent example of what they are referring to.

I'm Coming Out... With Cancer!

A few days later, after my immediate family was informed, I "Came out with Cancer" by sharing my diagnosis publicly. Emotionally, it was easier to tell extended family and friends all at once instead of individually. I created a social media cancer journal where I shared my journey with funny anecdotes to keep everyone updated and create awareness and hope, transforming my tragedy into humor.

The news spread like wildfire. While I did receive a lot of support from most people, I was also ghosted by others. Some simply disappeared as if cancer was contagious. I don't get it; I had cancer, not cooties. I guess cancer will scare some people away. A deadly illness is an excellent way to discover your real friends. Those friends are like bras—supportive, comfortable, and continually lift you.

Calm. Peace. Courage. Faith. Humor.

Having cancer is a lonely experience. You can't really ask anyone what to do. It can be a heavy burden on someone else, but my loved ones helped me find peace amidst this chaotic situation where everything seemed to be slipping through my hands. I tried playing the victim for one quick second, but their words of encouragement and trust in me made me realize I was a victor. They knew that I had the strength, courage, and attitude to fight it, and they would support me all the way. My family's encouragement gave me the willpower to get through to what I'd call the most dramatic phase of my life.

As sad as I was with this diagnosis, deep inside, I was relieved it happened to me and not to any of my children or family members. Who else could deal with this better than me? I mean, I am Superwoman, according to my family. Quite frankly, I doubt I would have had the strength to face this any other way. I knew myself, my strength, and my capabilities, and I was certain I would beat cancer.

---

*"You never know how strong you are
until being strong is the only thing you have."*
—Bob Marley

Through your trials, you will understand your strengths because, as the saying goes, "You never know how strong you are until being strong is the only thing you have." When confronted with difficulties, we have two choices: be passive and accept whatever is offered, or be active, informed, accept the support, and fight like hell. Adversities make us stronger and help us overcome our limits, and while we may not understand at the moment what the *blesson* might be, we must have faith and keep going. In the process, we will grow and gain confidence, resilience, determination, and the courage to overcome it.

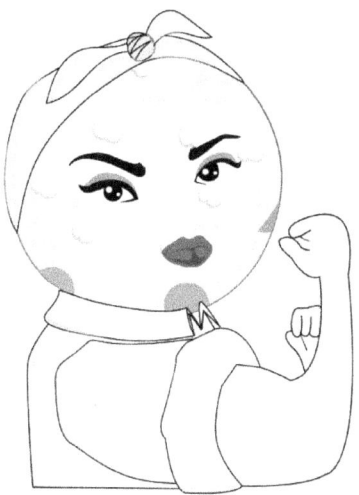

Tough Cookie

['ko͝okē] – Noun

1. Someone with just the right mix of sweetness and strength.

2. One who doesn't crumble under pressure.

3. A fighter who's too busy kicking butt to sit down and cry but knows it's OK to do both.

4. A person who doesn't always ask for support but has a lot of friends who would do anything to help.

—Unknown

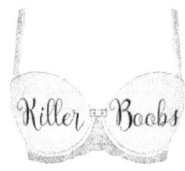

Chapter 3
My Boobs, First in Line

One in eight women gets breast cancer...
My boobs volunteered as tribute.

Cancer is just a word, not a sentence.

Before my diagnosis, cancer was just a word to me. Yes, I knew what it meant, but I never researched it. Why would I? It's not like it would ever happen to me. If you ask me today, I can explain my condition and everything about it in one single breath.

Surprisingly enough, I discovered that one in eight women is diagnosed with breast cancer, and of course, I am one. My boobs volunteered as tribute. I was quite offended by that decision. How dare they?

At this point, I had no choice but to put on my big girl pants and confront my cancer. Like the nerd I am, I sat down with a pen and a notebook to take notes as I spoke to the doctor over the phone. What is my diagnosis? How is it treated? What are my options? What doctors should I see? And the list went on and on.

My initial Diagnosis was *Stage Two Invasive Carcinoma Ductal.*

Now, I was even more offended at my boobs for taking it to the next level. Let's talk about beating cancer; I just beat stage one without any effort. Way to go!

As I continued to do the required generic testing, I learned that there are different types of breast cancer. My cancer was *Triple Negative Breast cancer*, a kind of breast cancer that is usually more aggressive, harder to treat, and more likely to come back. OK, now I was really perplexed. Triple-Negative? How ironic is it that you can be a super positive person and get a triple-negative diagnosis? Sure, you can; I just did! They say God doesn't give you more than you can handle, so He must think I am a badass.

With so much information and so many decisions to make, I called my sister, explained the diagnosis in detail, and got to work. The aggressiveness with which she and I did our research was impressive. We were more thorough than a detective at a crime scene, researching the best doctors, treatments, course of action, etc. We were ready, and at that point, we realized cancer was just a word, not a sentence.

Decision Time: Rock, Paper, Scissors

Like many women, I find it hard to make decisions. Something as simple as choosing a pair of shoes could be a challenge. So you can imagine my struggle to decide my best treatment options with decision-making skills closely resembling a squirrel crossing the street. I didn't know where to look. The more I researched, the more confused I got. Terms like lumpectomy, mastectomy, radiation, chemotherapy, and reconstruction were all gibberish to me.

After visiting many doctors to get a second, third, and even a fourth opinion, the diagnosis remained. Well, no! While talking to a fellow survivor and picking her brain on the subject, I discovered that I had been misdiagnosed and that my cancer was just at stage one. This was a huge sigh of relief! What else could the doctors have been wrong about? Maybe this cancer thing is not real? Wishful thinking. During those two weeks of doctor's visits, I felt like I was sharing my boobs with the world—flashing them every other minute. Hi Doctor, my name is Lucy, and these are my killer boobs!

Doctors Should be Like Bras... A Good Fit

Having cancer made me sensitive, vulnerable, and even skeptical. I couldn't trust my own boobs, let alone a new doctor. During the interview process, I came across some pretty harsh and blunt doctors. One, in particular, left me in complete distress. She was direct and had very little empathy. "Oh, you have triple-negative cancer. That is a very aggressive cancer. You are up for a tough ride. If this cancer comes back, you are done. We need to act quick!" Who the heck wants to hear that? While listening to her disheartening prognosis, I realized there were a few dead plants around the office. "Gee, I wonder why they died?"

If the plants had no chance, where would that leave me? I ran out of the office and was ready to quit before starting. I realized that, like some of my old bras, this doctor was not a good fit for me and my boobs. Thankfully, as I continued my search, I came across a team of doctors who took the time to listen, explain, and give me the encouragement and hope I needed to start my journey. Sometimes a doctor's comforting and reassuring words are the most potent medicine in times of distress.

Done Deal. Let the Cancer Ass-Kicking Begin!

After much consideration and deliberation with the crazy committee in my head, I came to peace with the following course of action: I would "Marie Kondo" my breasts with a bilateral mastectomy because I wanted no chance of finding another lump in the other boob. I already know they like to attack, and I don't want to deal with it again. Besides, having two boobs is overrated. The bilateral mastectomy also liberated me from radiation therapy, which was one less step to worry about. It's not like radiation treatment would make me any more radiant.

OK. Boobs situation resolved... a huge weight off my chest. Next!

Given that my tumor was small and was indeed only stage one, I was given the option to opt out of chemotherapy. However, due to the aggressiveness of my cancer, it was highly recommended to reduce recurrence, and like the badass that I am, I said, "Bring on the cocktail!"

While talking to my doctor, I asked, "Am I going to lose my hair?" I already knew the answer, but they say hope is the last thing you lose. "Yes," he replied, "You will lose a year of your life to gain the rest of your life." Well, that was somewhat comforting. I would have to suffer for one year to gain my life back. OK, if that is my only choice. The doctor gave me a plan and a sequence of events to follow, and I became an active partner with my doctor in this fight, giving me some control.

People are entitled to their own opinion but on their own boobs.

While some people find it helpful to ask for advice from friends and family, this was tricky for me because there were too many conflicting opinions.

"Don't you dare remove both of your breasts!"

"Do a single mastectomy. There is only one damaged boob."

"Skip the chemo; you don't need all those chemicals."

"A lumpectomy is your best choice."

"Opt for holistic medicine."

"Go Vegan! Try alkaline water, frozen lemon, essential oils, healing crystals, yoga…"

OMG, Stop! And shut the front door! These are my boobs, my body, and my cancer. I get it, everyone wants what's best for me, and of course, they are entitled to their own opinions and can make decisions about their own boobs. It's nice to know that I have an endless supply of advice when needed. Regardless of the different suggestions and opinions, I had made up my mind. I went with the decision that brought me peace and was best for my family and me. I will chop them off and get chemo! They tried to kill me first. The war was on.

In the meantime, this coupon would do:

Use the following card when necessary. For example, when someone tells you what you do with your killer boob.

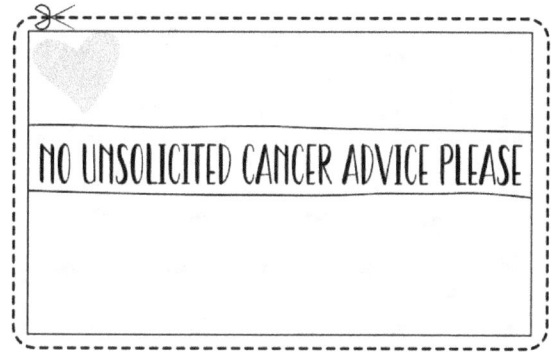

Understanding my diagnosis and considering the risks and benefits of the treatment I chose was extremely important to me. This allowed me to advocate for my own health and make informed decisions that kept me at ease. My sister was always on point, providing me with the necessary questions for every doctor's visit. She was so thorough that the doctors were impressed by "my knowledge." Yes, I took the credit for her research and felt proud. I felt smarter than a 5th grader.

My consultations with the doctors were more like interview sessions. A pen, paper, and a recorder were a must for each appointment because I did not want to miss a single thing. After being diagnosed with cancer, not only does your mind wander, but sometimes it leaves completely.

The Sisterhood of the Traveling Cancer

Never underestimate the power of a good support network. Finding a network of amazing women to help and support me through the process was vital for me. When you are diagnosed with cancer, you enter the Sisterhood of the Traveling Cancer. Here, everyone is ready to support you and share stories of hope, faith, and courage.

Through these women, I was able to find hope and courage to know that I would get through this and that I was not alone. Talking to these women comforted me and gave me peace.

Blesson: You can make a decision based on fear or faith.

We face challenges in life and must be ready to make difficult decisions that perhaps not everyone will agree with, and that's OK. Going through a trauma like cancer can make us vulnerable and cause us to question our choices. This is where faith comes in. "Faith is like Wi-Fi. It's invisible but has the power to connect you to what you need."

Taking the necessary steps even when the path was unclear and believing God would guide me through the process helped me feel at peace. It was time to stand up for myself and not get caught up in the people-pleasing game, especially from those who have not had killer boobs. No one could feel my pain, doubts, and uncertainty better than I did. So, who better than me to be at peace with my decisions?

I am a firm believer that attitude is everything. Cancer came to shake me and test my strength, but he failed to realize he messed with the wrong person because I was informed and determined. In my mind, I had only two options:

I CANsurvive or I CANsurrender.

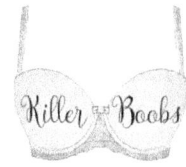

Chapter 4
Goodbye, Boobies

Goodbye and God Bless

The day of my mastectomy was bittersweet, actually more bitter than sweet. On the one side, I was going to take this *thing* off my chest, and on the other, my two boobs would be gone forever.

The surgery was scheduled for 1:00 pm, and my instructions were not to eat for at least six hours before surgery. That was a bit upsetting, considering I'm always hungry. In fact, I've never been so hungry in my entire life since the minute they told me I couldn't eat. My father, who came to visit me from New York for the first time, courtesy of cancer, woke up early to make me a delicious and filling breakfast. Cooking for and feeding his children has always made him happy. He wanted to ensure that at least my stomach was content before the surgery. I ate with no remorse; why bother counting calories when I was about to lose 10 lbs. of boobs?

My mom, siblings, husband, kids, and I gathered to say a prayer. We hugged as a symbol of unity, strength, and faith. "Goodbye, boobies, and God Bless. Off to heaven, you may go in peace."

I saw the worry in their eyes, especially my dad's. I had never seen him cry so much. He has always been known for his sense of humor, but that was as gone as my boobs were about to be. I was never a daddy's girl, but I felt like one at this moment. I wanted to go back in time and be the happy little girl who looked forward to my dad's storytelling. This story I was in was not fun.

Saying goodbye to my kids was really tough that morning. They were confused with everything that was happening. They did not go to school that day in observance of my boobs. Since my boobs had fed them for a few months each, this was their way of paying tribute.

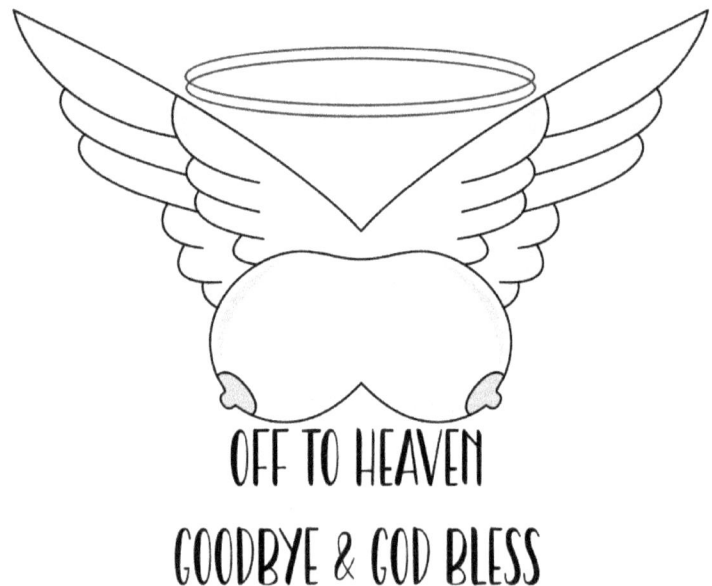

The Moment Has Come... Boobs be Gone!

My sister helped me pack my bag with all the post-mastectomy essentials: a special robe with internal pockets for the drains, flip-flops, loose clothes, a phone charger, and the first-class VIP ticket to the hospital. She was on top of her game. I felt as ready as an expectant mother leaving for the hospital to deliver her child, except I was going to deliver a silly tumor along with my incorrigible boobs.

OK, let's get this done! *"My boobies soon will be gone, but I will still rock on,"* I said in a funny tone. At least I got my family to chuckle. I sure know how to break the ice in a difficult situation. I am sure of two things: one, I had breast cancer, and two, I have an awesome sense of *humor.*

I was quiet on the drive to the hospital, reflecting and contemplating that my boobs would be gone soon. Deep inside, I was conflicted, nervous, and emotional, but for the sake of being a superwoman, I kept my composure.

"You've got this! You are going to be OK. You are like a phoenix; you rise from ashes!!!" I repeated to myself, activating my pep talk generator. My heart was pounding like a drum, but there was no turning back. I was ready, well, at least pretending to be. They say you need to *fake it until you make it,* and I was already practicing for the fake boobs to come.

After being admitted to the hospital, I changed into my hospital gown. I know these are typically not flattering, but I was rocking it. I've always had an excellent sense of style, and this occasion deserved no less. I even had time to take some selfies for the cancer fan club. The nurse ran some tests, placed the IV, and started the investigation process (well, at least that's what it felt like being asked so many questions). The room was cold, the air was thick, and the fear and anxiety were evident.

My family said goodbye and joined my friends in the waiting area. As the nurses prepared to transfer me to the operating room, my thoughts were all over the place, with more tabs open than an internet browser, not knowing where the music was coming from. Are you ready?" the nurse asked. "Yes!" I replied without hesitation, but with a cracked voice and tears rolling down my cheeks. They injected me with "*Happy Juice*" (the anesthesia). "God, you are in control," I prayed. I felt calm and happy, and off I went. Goodbye boobs, and God bless.

Knock, Knock, Who's There? Not my Boobs.

I woke up and thought, "I'm still here! It is a good day!" I was happy to see my family's joyful faces.

The tumor was removed along with 11 lymph nodes to ensure the margins were clear of cancer. "Look who's flat now," I said to my family, hoping to alleviate the tension. I felt lighter and had a good attitude since everything was off my chest. I looked down to see my nonexistent boobs. I was bandaged up like a mummy and couldn't see anything. The doctor had advised me that I would be as flat as a pancake, so I was expecting nothing more.

I wondered if having no boobs would at least make my butt look bigger; that's always a plus. To my surprise, when the bandages were removed, my boobs looked more like two fried eggs with a hard yolk. I had a little cushion. Oh, thank goodness! It's one thing to wish I had smaller breasts and another thing to have a chest as flat as an ironing board. Luckily, my incision was around the areola, so my nipple skin was left intact, which was a huge relief. I cannot imagine the distress I would have felt if my nipples had been gone.

In hindsight, I felt weird that my boobs were gone. My silhouette had changed; it was as if I had been reincarnated in a different body. I think I prefer big boobs after all!

My New Breast Friends

Is there such a thing as temporary boobs? Yes, I now had a pair, and they are called tissue expanders. I had never heard of such a thing until breast cancer decided to pay me a visit. These empty implants would be placed under the pectoral muscle to help the skin stretch and would be my breast friends for a few months until my chemo treatment was over. (I called them my "breast friends" to keep things cordial. Knowing my breasts are vengeful and dangerous, I needed to make them my allies.)

The expanders were the most uncomfortable and unattractive pair of boobs you can imagine. It looked like I had a boob job failure. They were hard and shapeless, making me feel like I had two flat, heavy rocks under my numb skin. For safety's sake, hugging was not an option.

My Boobs Editor

I was given a special remote to control my new breasts. The purpose was to gradually fill them with carbon dioxide through a port until I reached my desired breast size. Once my skin was stretched enough, I would be ready for reconstructive surgery with permanent implants. How cool is this amazing gadget? *I can inflate my breasts as much or as little as I want,* I thought to myself. It was like having a boob editor that would allow me to make adjustments as needed.

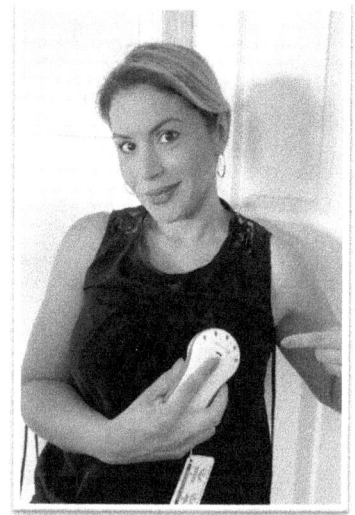

I was excited, knowing I would have complete control over the size of my boobs, and eager and ready to start. I felt like a kid in Toys "R" Us. (I still have it, if anyone is interested in having bigger boobs. I'm selling it to the highest bidder. Hurry!)

My Rebel Boob

Those of us who are mothers of more than one child can agree that there is always a rebel child in the group. I'm no exception. In addition to my rebel child, I also have a rebel boob. Yes, the killer boob, the one that has it out for me, the vengeful one! As happy as I was to control the size of my boobs, the excitement was cut short a month later. A few hours after pairing the remote and my boobs for the first time and filling them with the recommended amount of gas, I started feeling discomfort and tightness.

I felt like I had been hit by a truck and couldn't walk straight. I looked like the hunchback of Notre Dame. I figured this was normal while the muscle was being stretched, so I took it in like Wonder Woman. The pain persisted. A few days later, my rebel boob turned as red as a tomato and looked like it was ready to explode. The following day, I woke up drenched, leaking fluid like a sieve. "What is going on," I exclaimed! My breastfeeding days are long gone. I rushed to see the doctor, who immediately said I had an infection and an excess amount of liquid that needed to be extracted right away. He pulled out a needle longer than a skewer and immediately inserted it to deflate the boob. No anesthesia was required because my boobs were nonexistent, and the doctor was just pinching an empty implant surrounded by excess liquid. I was baffled, wondering what else this mischievous boob would do to get back at me. It was a cold war between us. She was indeed on a mission to kill me.

After that incident, I didn't want to expand them ever again. I was scared even to touch the boob editor. Eventually, I had no choice but to continue to expand the skin. I wish I could report that everything turned out well, but that was not the case. My rebel boob did it again. Something about that boob that just needs attention, and there I was, rushing to the doctor again with my swollen, ready-to-pop killer boob. After these incidents, the discomfort diminished; we made peace and continued our journey as breast friends.

Blesson: Who needs boobs with my funny personality?

The mastectomy changed me. I knew that having no boobs wouldn't make me disabled, but it would make me a bit unstable, at least for a while. Getting used to my new self-image was an adjustment. My body had been altered, and things were rearranged. Part of my femininity and motherhood was missing. My sensitivity was gone forever, something I would have to learn to deal with for the rest of my life. This is, without a doubt, life-changing, but I do not regret my decision. I made this choice in order to live. I do not feel like less of a woman. On the contrary, I am embracing this new version of myself. I feel confident and beautiful, and my scars symbolize my strength.

I woke up to a second chance and a new appreciation for life. A new beginning and a new perspective. Some women diagnosed with breast cancer aren't lucky enough to make it this far, but I did, with nipples and all. And for that, I am grateful and blessed. I lost a part of my body, but now I choose to count my blessings and focus on what I gained: resilience, courage, strength, and most importantly, my life, even without boobs.

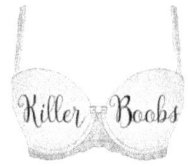

Chapter 5
One Cancer for All

In this family, no one fights alone.

It's been said that raising a child takes a village, but I say it takes a village to help a family member go through a life-threatening illness such as cancer. When my immediate family found out I had cancer, they all made plans to come to see me from New York. I didn't know whether to be happy or offended. My long-awaited family reunion was finally happening, courtesy of cancer. For the first time in thirteen years since I moved to Miami, I was able to gather them all together, even my divorced parents. Now, that was interesting; it was like having Hillary Clinton and Donald Trump in the same room, ready for a debate. Cancer is funny that way. For a few days, we were a united, happy family, cooking, eating, and watching TV together like the good old days. Well, except for my parents, who somehow managed to squeeze in a few debates—they had to keep the excitement going.

As the days passed, I noticed certain family members took their roles very seriously. They all became essential to this, and their unconditional support made the process seem a bit less traumatic.

Cancer Doesn't Come with a Manual; it Comes with a Warrior Mother

To say that my mother is a prayer warrior is an understatement. I'm sure she is the only person who doesn't have time to pray for herself because she is too busy praying for her children. Her faith is admirable. The second she learned I had cancer, she activated her prayer committee, who were on call 24/7. She did not doubt for one second that God was in control and that I would beat this cancer, which made me feel safe and confident. I knew she had a special connection with God and that He had my back. Florida became her new home; she left all her responsibilities behind to care for me wholeheartedly.

Her mission was to get me through this and ensure that I was well taken care of and, most importantly, well-fed. Oh boy! I already knew my diet would be altered. She is a great cook, not the healthiest, but definitely the tastiest. Nothing beats my mom's homemade meals. I wish I had that attribute. Knowing I had a special diet, she quickly adapted to my requests, at least for a while. I was in heaven. She also became a juicing guru, mixing veggies and fruits, wheatgrass, ginger, turmeric, apples, cranberry, and vodka. Oops, not the last one—wishful thinking. My mom's primary concern was ensuring my immune system was higher than the Empire State Building. She and God were on a mission to get me through this. I am 100% certain that her prayers did wonders.

My mom and I love each other, but we both have strong opinions, so we tend to bump heads from time to time. During my treatment, she became overprotective of me, making it challenging for me to go about my "normal" life.

Sometimes I would complain that she was invading my personal space, to which she would remind me that I came out of her personal space. Gosh, I wonder where I get my strong character from? She meant well, and her goal was for me to rest while she took care of my needs, but of course, I couldn't be still; I am always on the go, and cancer wasn't going to stop me. The truth is, I don't know where I would be without my praying and protective mother.

Her love and support are unconditional, and no matter the circumstances, she and God will always be there.

My Sister's Keeper

My sister and I are seven years apart, but we are like fat thighs—we always stick together. She is the one who keeps me grounded and calls me the minute I post a selfie on Instagram to point out that my toes are not aligned, or my shirt is a little wrinkled. She is the one who would pick me up if I fell—as soon as she stopped laughing. That's my sister!

I think she really loves me because her care and compassion are immeasurable. She has always protected me, even from getting in trouble with our mom in our younger years. This time was no different; she had my back. She became my keeper and held my hand as we went through this new adventure together. I get it, not everyone is lucky to have a bad-ass sister like me, and she was not going to let cancer come between us.

My sister lives about 1350 miles from me, but it felt as if she was right by my side every step of the way. She took this cancer thing personally and researched my alternatives thoroughly. Back off, cancer! My sister is in charge. I felt as proud as a peacock. She called numerous doctors, dealt with insurance issues, and formulated all the questions to ask. She even shaved her hair off in solidarity. Not really, that was just a joke. (It would have been nice.) Although she didn't shave her head, she did wear a head wrap and a wig for twinning purposes. She likes to be told she looks like me, and she does. We are like two peas in a pod, except she is much younger and friendlier! Ugh, rude!

Official Spokesperson

Cancer can be a touchy subject. Sometimes it's awkward to ask the person going through it, "Hey, how is your cancer going?" So, I needed a spokesperson, and my sister was a perfect fit for that role; she became my cancer representative. She was in charge of updating family and friends who wanted to stay informed about my medical updates. Some people were hesitant to approach me. I think they thought I was a bit intimidating, and they were probably right. You would be too if someone had chopped off your boobs. Besides, she was always the friendlier one, so it worked out great.

Giving up is not an option when you have two beautiful children who call you "Mommy."

Cancer was an abstract concept to my children. They didn't fully understand what was going on. That didn't surprise me, though, because I didn't understand what was happening myself. We were all lost in Cancerville, wherever that is. They had to adapt to their mom being sick, pale, and bald as a coot.

We tried to keep their routines as normal as possible, not to alter their lives. My three-year-old son continued his life as usual. He is such a happy and clever little boy who only cares about playing and food, just like his mother. "The apple doesn't fall far from the tree," they say. My daughter was a bit older, and although not quite sure about everything that was going on, she knew her mother was not well. She is as sweet as a pie, loving, caring, and has a great disposition to help. She wanted to help me in any way she could, so she gave me my meds, applied my scar cream religiously every night, and ensured I was always comfortable. She was only seven, but she acted like she was seventeen. She definitely takes after me.

Cool Mom Fighting Cancer

After I recovered from phase one of the fight—the mastectomy—and entered phase two—chemo—I became their cool mom fighting cancer. We always had an agenda filled with activities. We went on a few trips to Disney (yes, again!), the zoo, the beach, and tons of other fun places. I'm not sure if it was to keep my kids entertained or to let my inner child have fun. We managed to stay busy and have a blast. Let me just add that my overprotective mother was not so happy about this. She feared that I would have an adverse reaction by being so exposed, and of course, I did.

My killer boob retaliated again. I developed an infection, leaving me no choice but to stay in bed for a few days. I hate it when my mom is right! "Mothers know best," they say. Her desire was for me to remain in bed resting, but I refused. I was being a rebel, like my killer boob. I wanted to be a cool mom, have fun, live like cancer was not controlling my life, and spend time with my kiddos. My kids kept things in perspective and kept me going. Their outpouring of love, laughter, and affection gave me the motivation and strength to continue the fight. How could I give up with two beautiful children who call me mommy?

My Fight was His Fight

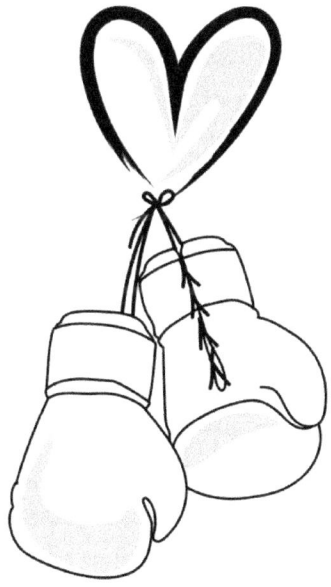

My husband was the strongest one of all. I can't tell you how he felt about this cancer thing because he has always been calm and quiet, but he was there, like my rock! He was supportive and ready to fight because my fight was his fight, and there was no question about it. He went to every doctor's appointment and chemotherapy session. This was interesting at times because my husband was always next to me as I flashed my boobs to an arsenal of male doctors. Awkward! But he was there like white on rice. His life shifted as much as mine. He had to readjust and take on all the household and business responsibilities. Getting us through this was his main objective. He never disagreed with any of my medical decisions. Why would he? I am the woman, and I'm always right!

He was a provider and would go out of his way to buy anything I needed during my treatment: the best water, the most organic vegetables, the best juicer, a special pillow, food cravings, trips to Disney, and a new Chanel bag. Oh, wait! He missed that last thing. It would have been nice, though. I'm still wondering why I didn't ask for one. It must have been the chemo brain. The point is that he was there for me during this traumatic time, reassuring me that I was going to be well. He always thought I had superpowers to solve problems and not let anything or anyone intimidate me, not even cancer.

The Cancer Crosscheckers

In addition to my amazing support at home, I also had a group of family and friends helping me that I referred to as "Team Lucy." They made sure all my bases were covered and cross-checked: babysitting, driving my kids to and from school, bringing me food, cleaning my house, coming up with fun things to do, making me laugh, throwing me a party, going to my chemo sessions, and even helping me choose flattering wigs. My team was the best, and it continued to grow as my treatment progressed. People whom I would have never predicted showed their support in different ways. Some sent me encouraging gifts, and others came to visit me. How blessed was I? They really came through. It is true what they say, friends don't let friends fight cancer alone. I don't know how I would have done it without their help and constant cheerleading. They were certain that with their support, cancer had picked the wrong team to mess with.

> **Blesson: Be kind to yourself and have a good support system.**

My family and friends may have been unable to prevent me from getting cancer, but they made sure I didn't face it alone. Going through cancer could be lonely because no one can understand your pain and the rollercoaster of emotions you are feeling. Some days feel as if you are on a bipolar express train. One minute, you are riding a magical unicorn on an emotional rainbow; the next, you feel like demons are eating your soul in the darkness. It was hard, but I was blessed to have a strong emotional support system that allowed me to focus on my healing. I realized three things:

1. My support system is stronger than an army.

2. I am a strong woman because a strong woman raised me.

3. Anything is possible when you have the right people by your side.

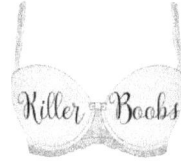

Chapter 6
Thanks for the Mamories

> *"Life may not be the party we hope for,
> but while we are here, we shall dance."*
> —Jeanne C. Stein

My mastectomy day was approaching, and I wanted to give my boobs a proper farewell. They were about to embark on a voyage of no return, and I needed to show them my appreciation. I realize they were killer boobs, but they were my killer boobs, and I was grateful for all they had done for me for thirty-nine years. This party served two purposes: (1) to pay tribute to my boobs and (2) to reassure myself and my loved ones that I would be OK. "This too shall pass," I said to the crowd in my joking voice. "Probably like a kidney stone, but it will pass." Uplifting them was my own uplift. I knew a positive attitude would not cure my cancer, but it would annoy my killer boobs, and that made it worth it.

My friends all came dressed in pink as a tribute to my boobs. Everyone had a blast at the party. We laughed, cried, took pictures, and even sang Karaoke, something I love to do. Funny enough, one of my favorite go-to songs has always been "I will survive," which was perfectly suited for the occasion. My family and friends celebrated me, and for the first time in a long time, I celebrated my boobs. They had their own theme cake, and it was amazing. I felt showered with love and support. My boobs deserved it. I was mean to them and unhappy with their size, but they still hung in there. They were sad for a while, and I was the culprit, so they tried to kill me to get revenge. I am happy to report that we made peace before we said goodbye. We had a heart-to-heart conversation in front of my bedroom mirror; I apologized, took pictures to immortalize them, and thanked them for the *mamories.*

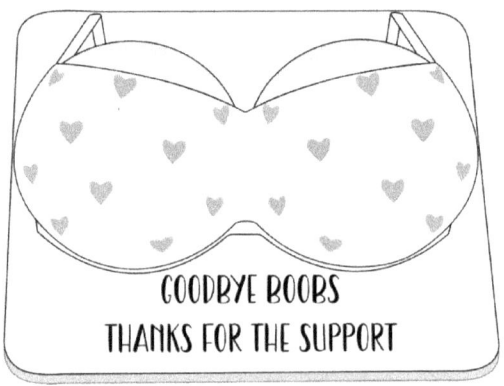

Cancer Fabulous & Forty

It was two days before I started my chemo treatments, and my 40th birthday was in a few days. Wow, the timing for this could not have been better—what a way to celebrate. I guess the only cocktail I would be having was the chemo. *I wonder if I could add a slice of lime to it,* I thought to myself. My friends and my husband threw me a birthday party, and since I am a party queen, I couldn't have been happier. I was ready to celebrate my Fabulous 40th. Deep down, there was a slight fear that this could be my last one. With cancer, you never know what the outcome will be. However, I did not want to allow the negative thoughts in my head to rule. Instead, I cleared my mind of any crazy thoughts to enjoy my well-planned party.

This birthday party was one for the records. The food, drinks, décor, and people were perfection. There was even a live band. I felt special and could not have asked for a better party. Once again, my friends and husband outdid themselves. I felt blessed and happy and danced like nobody was watching because "*Life may not be the party we hope for, but while we are here, we should dance."*

Keep Calm and Find a Bomb Wig

Let's talk about hair! Depending on their treatment and type of cancer, some women are lucky enough not to lose their hair, but not me, of course. I did not qualify for that prize. Remember, God thinks I am a badass. My hair loss was inevitable. I tried opting for a cooling cap treatment, a very cold cap placed on the head while getting the chemo to prevent or reduce hair loss. However, with triple-negative cancer, not one single hair follicle in my body would survive. Now that was a hard pill to swallow. Hair has always been so important to me. It is part of a woman's femininity and a reflection of our identity. I guess at this point, my one and only choice was a wig. A Bomb Wig.

I went on a mission to find the perfect wig. Oh yes! I am vain like that. I took this as an opportunity to rock different looks and have fun with it. I gathered some of my "Team Lucy" gals and went in search of a wig. My first experience was a complete failure. The stylist knocked down every wig I chose and instead suggested ones that made me look like a traumatized eighty-year-old lady. He claimed that those were perfect for me.

I'm not sure what he was implying. I know chemo tends to age people, but I had not even started the treatment. I still looked my age. I should have known better; he looked like a rocker from the '80s. I refused to buy any of the wigs suggested and opted to buy a head wrap, which would probably look better than any of those antique wigs I tried on. I walked out of there sadder than a bride, unable to find her perfect wedding dress. I felt hopeless. They were supposed to be the wig experts, and I was sure I would find a cool wig there.

Since I am not one to give up easily, I continued my hunt. My girl gang and I visited several other places, and this time things were different. I tried different hair lengths, colors, and styles; I was having a blast, and my sister and friends joined me in trying different looks. We felt like Beyonce, except we were not the single ladies; I was more like the cancer lady. After a few outings searching for wigs, I finally found the one, the BOMB wig that made me feel like me. I knew it was the one. We just clicked! Now I was ready. Bring on the chemo!

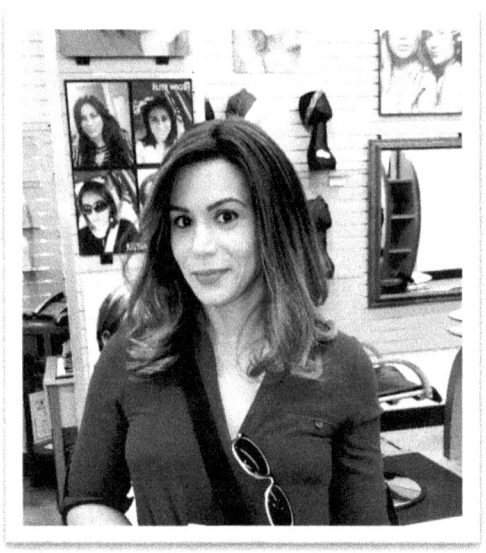

The Bomb Wig

Enough with the Celebrations. It was Time for the Real Cocktails: Chemo Cocktails.

It was time for the complete body poison. I'm not sure I was completely ready, except for my wig; that part was covered. The point is that I had to do it. The first step was undergoing minor surgery to insert the chemo port, a small silicone tube attached to the vein to administer the chemo. An incision was made on the right side of my chest, leaving me with another scar sponsored by cancer. I'm still wondering why this port isn't wireless with all of the advances in medical technology. I need some answers!

Step two was to attend a chemo orientation class, which is very appropriate for someone who is about to be completely disoriented. Before that class, I was prescribed a plethora of medications that I needed to bring with me to class to learn how to administer them properly. These pills were going to help prevent the potential side effects of the chemo. OK, let's go. I grabbed my bag full of drugs, and I was ready for my training. Like the nerd that I am, I also brought my notepad to take notes to ensure I didn't forget any instructions.

My daily medications included steroids, anti-nausea, pain killers, laxatives, antacids, sleeping pills, and pills for cramps, joint pain, and allergies. Oh my Gosh!! This was all to counteract the side effects of the chemo that gave the effect in the first place. Ugh. Why can they all be combined in one convenient dose? Or better yet, why aren't there any good side effects from all these pills? Like extreme sexiness or severe rejuvenation?

During orientation, my brain was like the Bermuda triangle. All the information went in, but it was never found. All I retained was:

> Every day before waking up, after dinner, before food, to be taken before bed, four times a day, three times daily, take one, or two or three.

Warning: For best results, follow the instructions you have been given exactly.

Please help! How am I supposed to keep up with this? Well, my ingenious sister came to the rescue! She came up with a plan. Of course, she did! She was always one step ahead of my cancer. She was, indeed, my keeper. She set an alarm for every single medication needed. It felt like an alarm was going off every five minutes. Sometimes I wanted to hit the snooze button and wake up a year later, be done with cancer, and have a new pair of perky boobs. I managed to keep up and follow through as directed. Chemo was the next stop.

Blesson: Attitude is everything, so pick a good one.

Sometimes special moments bring happiness to our lives and give us hope. I knew the worst days of my life were approaching, and things were going to change drastically in Cancerville. I did not want to give the negative committee in my head a voice. I tried to make the best of it with the best attitude and disposition. I always tried to have fun and see the positive in every situation, no matter how difficult. Dancing, singing, putting a smile on my face, and rocking a bomb wig would show cancer that I was ready for the fight and determined to win. I had been warned that this would be a tough voyage, but I approached it with a positive attitude. The parties, the wig outings with my girls, and the chemo classes were all part of a plan that I decided would be entertaining and humorous. After all, cancer took my boobs, not my sense of humor.

Five Tips for Getting Through Cancer

From a Badass Cancer Fighter

1. **Stay the course:** Maintain your routine as normal as possible. Don't let cancer anxiety consume you.

2. **Be informed and speak up:** You owe it to yourself and your loved ones to advocate for the treatments, doctors, and alternatives you feel comfortable with.

3. **Write it all down:** Track your symptoms, feelings, emotions, medications, questions and concerns for doctors, etc. Let it all out!

4. **Get a support system:** Find a network of doctors, fellow survivors, family members, and friends to help you and uplift you.

5. **Don't let cancer stand in your way:** Allow yourself a few days to cry and be scared. Then, roll up your sleeves, get your facts straight, and beat the heck out of cancer.

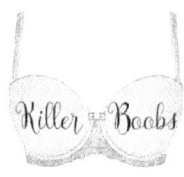

Chapter 7

Can You Add Some Tequila to That Cocktail?

Chemo sucks, but it does suck the cancer out of you.

Yay, chemo day! said no one ever.

It was Monday, the first day of my five-and-a-half months-long journey. I elected to do my treatments on Mondays, so the side effects of chemo would be over by the weekend. I have always been a good planner, even for chemo. I woke up early and had a great breakfast (screw the diet). I popped all the pills as instructed and, most importantly, prepped the port on my chest area. The instructions were to rub Lidocaine, numbing cream, on the area an hour before treatment, and I sure did. I did not want to feel a thing. It would have been great to have numbing cream for my brain. With my mother and husband, I arrived at the hospital with a bag filled with snacks, a blanket, a book, and water as if it was my first day of class. The moment has come.

The nurse did some blood work and took my vital signs. Everything was on point with me, except for the cancer. Other than that, I was perfect. I was taken to the infusion suite; it was time to access my port to start prepping for the infusion. The nurse wore gloves and a mask, and I also had to wear them.

I would have never thought we were secretly preparing for COVID season, which would happen a few years later.

My hands were shaking, my heart was pounding, and my emotions were all over the place. I knew this would change my life forever, but I wasn't sure how. The nurse had me take a deep breath so they could access the port. I had nothing to worry about, that area was numb, or so I thought. She inserted the port, and at that precise moment, I felt like I was being stabbed with a dagger, and my soul was about to pop out.

What just happened? What was the point of the numbing cream? I asked myself in complete discomfort—good question, especially if you rub it in the wrong area. Well, how was I supposed to know; it's not like I was paying attention during chemo orientation class when the process was explained to me. I could see that we were off to a great start.

Have You Ever Met the Devil? Well, I Sure Have!

Let me introduce you to the one and only Devil, the very RED DEVIL. Due to my type of cancer (triple-negative), my treatment consisted of two types of chemotherapy: Doxorubicin, also known as the "RED DEVIL" due to its effectiveness and adverse reactions, and Taxol, which supposedly would be a breeze. As you can imagine, just from that peculiar name that I refuse to repeat because even my tongue burns just by thinking about it. This was a killer chemo.

I had four long infusions of that diabolic liquid and twelve of the Taxol, the less harsh option. The Oncologist recommended I start with the "less harsh" one so my body could get used to the chemo. Of course, I didn't follow that advice; I wanted to get that "Red Devil" over and done with. Nothing with that name had room in my body, so I opted to kick the devil's butt. God was with me, and I would not fail. If I did, my mom would handle it with Him directly.

Straight out of Chemo

My first session was done. What a relief! I made it. I'm still alive. I felt like my head was filled with air, but I guess I was now less cancer-y than the day before. The first day was a walk in the park, Jurassic Park! I was sent home to rest with an injectable device, *Neulasta*, attached to my belly that would release a medication 24 hours later to keep my white blood cell counts up and avoid infections. Great, now I looked like a drugged and puzzled ex-convict with a GPS attached. This was getting better by the minute; not only was I fighting cancer, but also the Devil—the very red Devil. It was so red that my pee looked like tomato juice. As the day progressed and the chemo and the steroids kicked in, I had more energy than a child at bedtime. I was secretly hoping this device would give me superpowers. Why not? My family already thought I was Wonder Woman.

Let's Get Some Cocktails on Mondays

After finishing my first chemo, I shared it on social media, making a funny post about my first day of chemo, inviting friends and family to join me as I enjoyed some chemo cocktails on Mondays. I promised to add some lime to their cocktails. To my surprise, the outpouring of support was endless. Soon my Mondays became something to look forward to, not because of chemo but because of my gatherings, which helped me forget about the chemo effects. I was constantly surprised by family and friends from out of town who traveled to spend the day with me at my suite. Team Lucy became bigger and more fun. When they saw me walk in, the nurses at the infusion center would exclaim, "*Yup, it's Monday; it's party time. Team Lucy is in the house.*" They never said so, but I know they miss my gatherings.

My Monday get-togethers included laughter, reminiscing, encouragement, and most importantly, lots of love and support. It was the perfect prescription to cope with my cancer.

What? Chemo Will Kill the Hair Follicles in my Armpits?

Two weeks later, and just as expected, the inevitable started happening. My hair started falling out in chunks. Even my armpits, just in case you are wondering! This was devastating. I knew it was going to happen, but I didn't realize it would be so shocking. "*Let's just get this over with,*" I said to myself. I went to the salon to get a really short pixie cut. I figured I would rock that look until the hair was all gone.

The stylist prepared to cut my hair by washing it first. Little did I know that my scalp was super sensitive, and as soon as he washed my hair, most of it would be left in the shampoo bowl. I returned to the stylist's chair in complete despair. I wasn't prepared for this; I did not bring my bomb wig, hair wrap, or even mask to hide my face. Help! I didn't know whether to cry, scream, or die. I was in a rush to leave because I didn't want to be seen. I ignored everyone who wanted to talk, comfort me or ask me questions.

As I left to go home, I realized it was time to pick my kids up from school. OMG, this is going to be a shock. Would they even recognize me? I don't even recognize myself.

As soon as they saw me, they were in awe. "*Mommy, what happened to your hair?* They asked. I explained that this was part of the cancer process and that I was ok. The look on their face was frantic. I needed to get them something to eat, so we went to the closest pizza place. As we parked and got out of the car, my daughter questioned, "Mommy, are you getting out of the car looking like that?" Holy moly, she was embarrassed, and so was I. Kids are so honest. "Yes," I said very calmly, even though inside I wanted to scream and pull my hair out. Oh wait, I only had about five or six strands left, perhaps this was not a good idea.

We went inside quickly, ordered a pizza to go, and jetted out of there. As we approached our home, my son, who had not said a word as he must have been contemplating the scenery, exclaimed, "Mom, I don't like your hair like that. please put it back." Oh my, once again, I wanted to dig a hole and disappear. Sure, I replied. Thanking God for the Bomb wig I got.

My scalp was so sensitive that I couldn't wear the wig yet. Instead, I put a wrap around my almost completely bald little head. That was a very sad day for me. A few days later, I asked my husband to shave the remaining hairs on my head, and he honored my request. I felt like a different person—with two hard rocks on my chest and no hair on my head. I was officially ready for my bomb wig, but first, a picture.

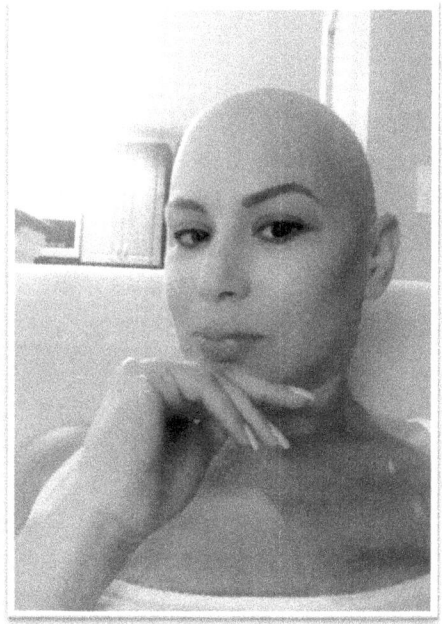

No Hair, Don't Care.

Since there is never a dull moment, or should I say a bald moment, I decided that I wanted to do a photo shoot. I figured this was the only time I would rock the bald look in my lifetime, so why not immortalize it? A dear friend put me in contact with a photographer, and she immediately agreed to take the photos. We set up a date, I found a glittery dress, arranged to get my makeup done, and voila! I was ready!

My makeup artist and my photographer outdid themselves. They were so accommodating and refused to accept any payment. They wanted me to feel like a Queen. Without hair, a queen is still a queen. Well, a chemo Queen. Their compassion, selflessness, and my rollercoaster of emotions had me in tears. Good thing for the waterproof mascara; it came in handy. I was all glammed and glittery, but my scalp felt naked and cold. Now I understand why newborn babies wear hats. As a matter of fact, my level of respect for bald men just went up.

The Shoot

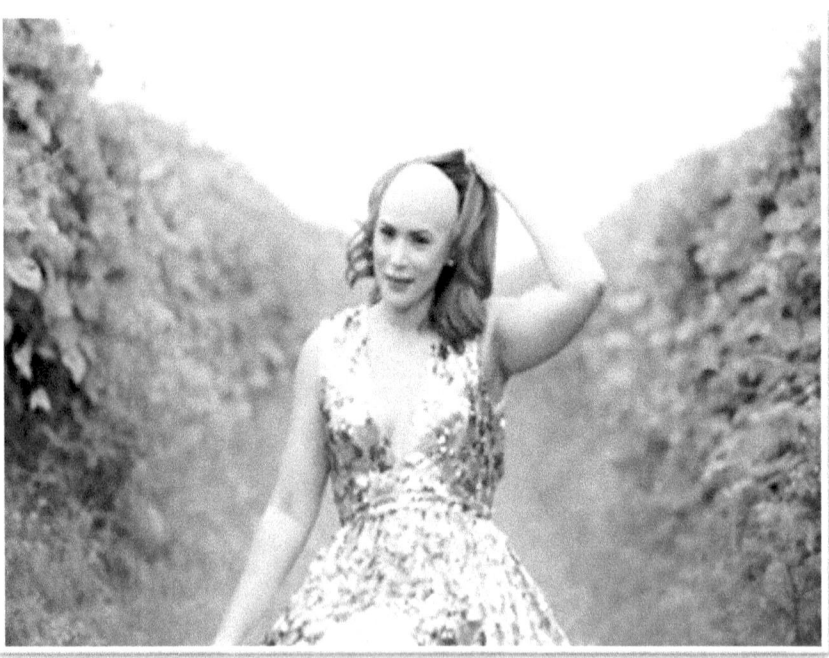

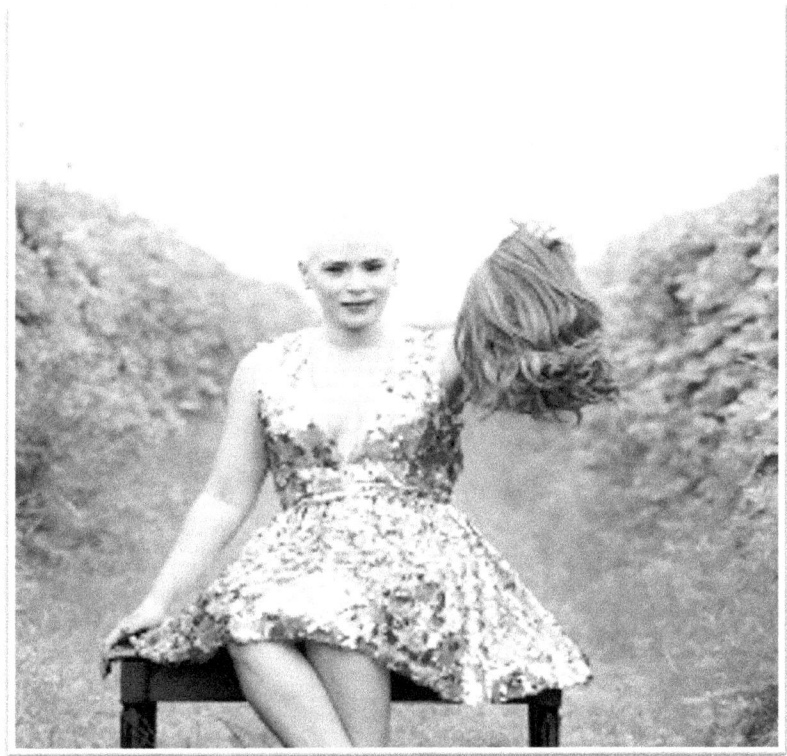

It Got Super Cold in Cancerville.

Ice, Ice, baby! "You must dip your hands and feet on ice for the entire duration of the infusion," the doctor said. "This will prevent neuropathy." "Neuropa-what?" Weakness, numbness, and nerve damage caused by chemo. Great! One more hurdle to jump. Now my chemo sessions consisted of not only infusions, but also two buckets filled with ice for my hands and feet.

It was now really cold in Cancerville, but I stayed the course. Some of my family members did it with me for support. Not really, but at least long enough to take pictures. It's the thought that counts.

Some of my Chemo Issues from head to toe:

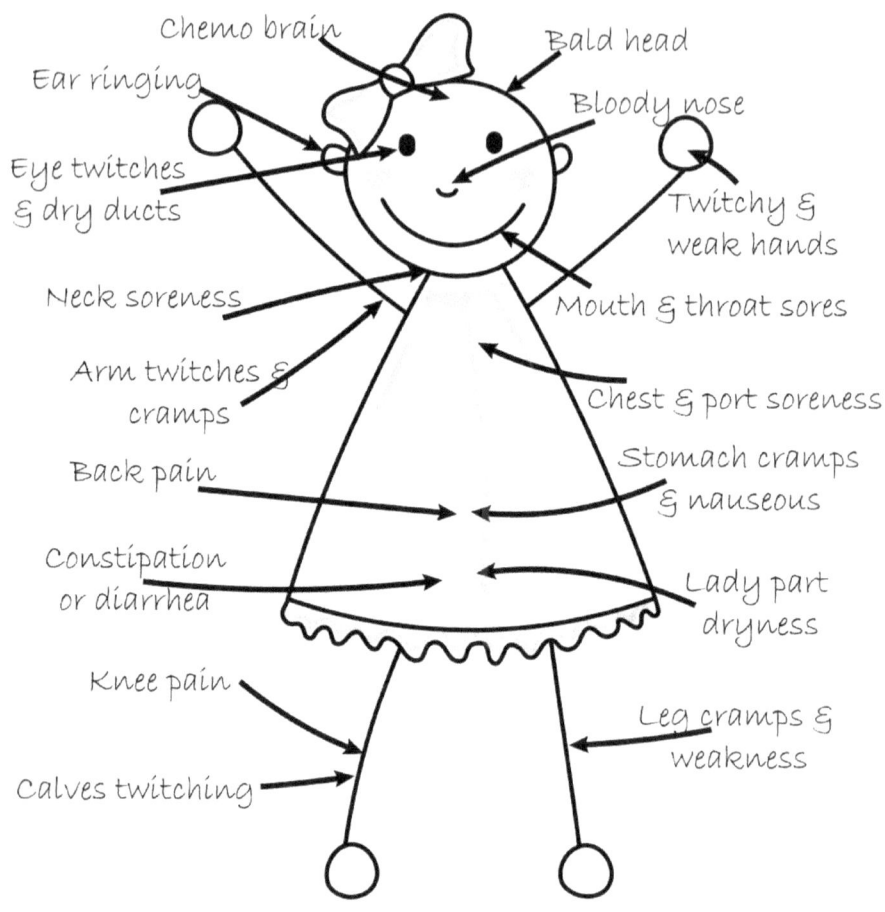

Fun stuff... But I got this!

If You Can't Beat 'em, Join 'em.

After a few months of chemo sessions, I was getting used to cancer. I could predict my week pretty well and control it. My weekly schedule was as follows:

Mondays Ready as a bullet to kill any possible cancer cell still in my body. Drowsy at first, but my energy thermometer would start rising.

Tuesdays With more energy than the energizer bunny, I can go on and on. Limitless energy and endurance. My best day of the week.

Wednesdays As tired as a bear during hibernation. Energy levels slowly decreasing, and the aches and pains started to appear.

Thursdays As useless as the "G" in lasagna. 104% tired and in a lot of pain. Not my best days.

Fridays Melancholic. Trying to control and convince the committee in my head that everything was going to be OK, and I must remain strong.

Saturdays Lethargic as a drunk turtle dozing under a sunflower after ingesting a bottle of valium. I did not feel like doing anything!

Sundays Whatever attitude. Get out of bed and make it to the sofa, but not playing an active role, just going with the flow to recover and start my week all over again.

Superhero Note

Chemo and recovery became the primary focus in my life but staying active was also important. Having things to look forward to and keeping busy helped distract me during my stay in Cancerville. I wanted to enjoy my good days with friends and family.

Funny enough, this is how I was perceived by some of my family members:

Excerpt shared from a family chat:

August 30th, 2018

We just got off the phone with Marvel and DC comics; we found their missing superhero! Her name is Lucy Beato, the queen of precious stones known to fight evil with beauty, humility, and optimism. Six months ago, our cousin/resident superhero, Lucy, was invited to a duel against breast cancer. Newsflash, she wins. We'll give you a snapshot of a typical day with Lucy.

So, Chemo Monday: We wake up 45 minutes late – she's up, our breakfast was ready, the coffee is brewing, kids have already been dressed and fed, and the eldest is off to school. So, we know Beyoncé woke up like that but turns out Lucy also wakes up looking flawless. Eyebrows on fleek; hair on point; and perfectly manicured nails. We pack into the car, half-asleep, in our wrinkled outfits, and she is driving through Florida traffic, with her hair flowing through the wind, unbothered. First stop – dropping her 3-year-old off at daycare. Second stop – dropping off her car at the (auto shop).

Next, we are off to chemo.

She takes a seat, and the four-hour duel begins.

Not once did she stop shining.

First – she offers snacks and coffee.

Second – she asks the nurse how she is doing and proceeds to explain how things will go, she could tell we were a little frazzled.

She entertains us with humorous childhood anecdotes, and before we know it, the match is over; we collect our belongings, and she invites us to lunch!

After having lunch, we track back to daycare and school and then head back home, where she makes us each a delicious latte and helps her kids with homework.

Lucy then decides we should all go out for ice cream! (It was amazing!)

It's bedtime again, the kids are all in their beds, and we just sit there in awe.

The next morning, we find our superhero brewing coffee, making breakfast, and tackling the day all over again!

> "I'm not saying that I'm Superwoman, but you've never seen me and Superwoman in the same room at the same time."

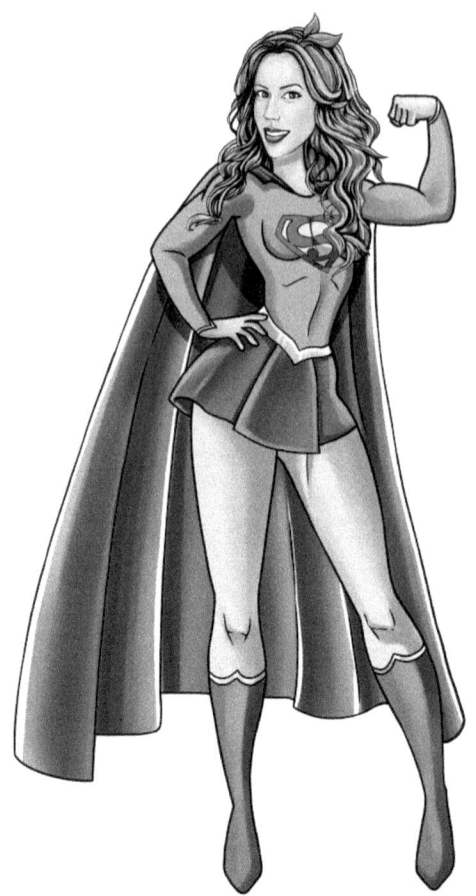

Blesson: Chemo warrior—I killed cancer cells one cocktail at a time.

I had a love/hate relationship with chemo for six long months, but it was time to break up and move on. It was my chemo graduation, which was kind of a big deal. Although I have graduated several times, this time was special. Nothing had ever felt more rewarding than my chemo graduation. I must admit that there were days I wanted to drop out of "The University of Hard

Knocks," but I didn't. I completed my cancer degree with honors and perfect attendance. I was proud. I fought, and I won.

That day was one for the records. No more needles, blood work, steroids, or ice baths. Cancer does not live here anymore; I beat it! Yes! I am a cancer warrior. Some of my friends and family were there to celebrate the grand finale when I would finally get to ring the bell and run like hell in celebration of my victory.

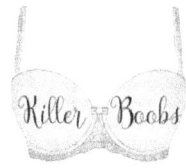

Chapter 8
A Boss Lady Fighting Cancer

"Running a business while going through cancer is easy; it's like riding a bike except the bike is on fire, with no seat, flat tires, and you're on fire."

—Medium Black Lined Journal

Managing a hair salon while fighting cancer was quite challenging. As a co-owner, my many roles included handling the day-to-day operations and finances, effectively leading a team, dealing with customers, hiring staff, serving coffee, sweeping the floors, washing the bowls, cleaning the toilets, etc. You know, the many hats of entrepreneurs.

It's a lot of work and very stressful, but also fun, glamorous, and rewarding. Nothing beats watching women feeling powerful while being pampered and as they get their hair styled and nails manicured. While all this could be enjoyable, running my business during this phase of my life was like trying to hold my hair together with one bobby pin—nearly impossible without a good grip. I had to think of something quick. Time was of the essence, cancer was not going to wait, and my business needed to continue running despite the circumstances. The show, or should I say, "the beauty," needed to go on. Clients and employees were counting on me, and I could not let them down.

To Tell or Not to Tell?

Once I had a definitive prognosis and a course of action for my treatment, I had to create a contingency plan to ensure the salon would continue to run smoothly. At first, I kept the news to myself because I did not want to put the business at risk by creating uncertainty amongst the staff. I needed to keep my composure and have the courage and strength to reassure my staff that everything would be OK.

I immediately started training my support staff to lead the team effectively. I hired a bookkeeper to track all the financial transactions properly, something I usually handled. Once the important things were taken care of, I told my key employees about my diagnosis and asked for their support. They immediately showed empathy and assured me everything would be just fine while I was away. I felt relieved and comforted knowing my staff would have my back and were committed to the company. Off to Cancerville I went.

Let it Go, Let it Go

Delegating has always been difficult for me; not because I don't appreciate the help, but because I feel no one does tasks as quickly and effectively as I can. I admit that is a terrible way of thinking. We all have flaws. As a consequence, I ended up doing everything myself, leaving me exhausted. Some days, I woke up so tired that the bags under my eyes were bigger than my boobs, which I've already shared with you that I felt were huge.

I hate to admit it, but I was a true perfectionist with acute attention to detail, but that behavior is all part of my past. When dealing with cancer, you don't have control of anything, let alone a business. I only needed to be a perfectionist when beating cancer. This was truly the time to let it go and trust that my team would work to the best of their abilities and that the business would continue to run effectively in my absence. I had no other choice. I wonder if delegating my worries would have worked?

Cancer, Please Just Send the Hot Mess Express Train to Take Me

When I asked, *can things get any more complicated?* It was a rhetorical question, not a command. While I was focusing on fighting cancer, our business rental lease expired, and we had to make some decisions. Everything was happening at once. You know that moment when you are at the edge of having a mental collapse, and then you're faced with one more minor inconvenience. *Cancer, please just send the hot mess express train to take me,* I thought. What am I going to do? I'm in the middle of a serious fight and can't afford to lose my life or my business.

My team and I immediately started brainstorming about our options and, luckily, were able to move the business right next door. However, this meant building a salon from scratch in just four months. How do you do that? Well, Superwoman to the rescue.

I hired a salon consultant to do all the negotiations and a general contractor to do the construction and deal with all the legal aspects (permits, etc.). I was on the phone constantly directing and overseeing the project to ensure it was going as planned. I felt half-dead and had very little energy, but things needed to get done, and cancer was not going to get in my way because I had a business to run.

Things to do Today: 1 Run a business 2. Beat cancer 3. Stay calm.

Nothing was going as it was supposed to. The timing was off, the contractor did not deliver, and the landlord was being difficult. At this point, if I had to rate my stress level, I would say I was pretty close to Britney Spears in 2007 when she shaved her head. Wait, my head was also shaved, so that makes sense. Still, I needed to stay calm. I was not beating cancer to die from stress. I had to focus on my final destination while readjusting my GPS to recalculate my route. Finally, we were able to move to the new location. It wasn't perfect, but at least the business kept running without interruptions.

At that point, I was almost done with chemo and soon would need to go back to work a few days a week.

A New Beginning

Coming back to work was interesting. The "new me" was different. Many of our regular clients did not know I was battling cancer, so seeing the new chunky and beaten me was a bit shocking. Before cancer, I was always thin and well put together, so the change was noticeable. Customers would say things like "You look so different" or "You have put on some weight." In my head, that meant, "You look like an overweight, half-dead zombie."

The comments always made me feel bad, but I would usually make a funny remark to lighten the mood. Any harsh remark can be softened with humor, which is my specialty. I was not going to allow those remarks to distract me or make me emotional; I was on a mission. Once I fully emerged in work, I felt more in control and more like myself. I put on my lipstick, my wig, and heels to finish beating cancer like a boss.

The Support Squad

Coincidence… I think not! At the hair salon, we have always supported the breast cancer foundation. Why that particular cause when there are so many others? Great question! Well, since there are no coincidences, it's either a message or a clue to a facet of our lives that requires attention. Every October, we created awareness with cancer-related events, such as a cut-a-thon, special promotions, raffles, and donations to raise money to support the cause. God works in mysterious ways. He wanted me to be involved as much as I could with the sisterhood of the traveling cancer community because he knew I would need the alliance. He was preparing me. Nice play, God. Love ya!

This year, of course, was not the exception, but it was different; cancer had hit home. Now the cause was even more symbolic. My staff outdid themselves, creating awareness, decorating, and planning a fundraiser. We even had special pink shirts that said "Team Lucy, Stronger Together." It was a special month filled with empathy, compassion, team cohesiveness, and awareness. We celebrated my victory. I felt really supported by my staff and wonderful clients. I will forever be grateful.

Blesson: I beat Cancer in heels.

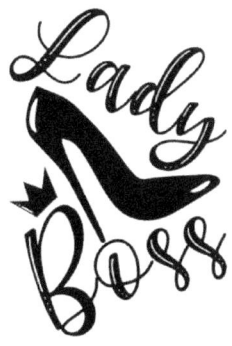

I did not have time to deal with cancer when I had a business to run and decisions to make. Carrying on as a businesswoman was important to me and kept me busy. So, I continued to work as much as I was able to and beat cancer wearing heels while learning a few *blessons* along the way.

First, my resilience and ability to withstand pressure are greater than what I gave myself credit for. I was able to overcome the unexpected and keep going.

Although I know that I am capable of doing many tasks, I realized I couldn't do everything myself. Asking my team for their help and support was vital for my business to continue thriving during this crisis.

Finally, my greatest *blesson* of all was learning to let go of the things I cannot control and asking God to take over. He always has control of any situation, despite how difficult it may seem. Since it all worked out for the best, I will, without a doubt, always "Let go and let God."

I am not beating cancer to die from stress.

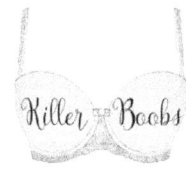

Chapter 9
Fighting Chemons and My Multiple Personalities

The good thing about multiple personalities is that if you collect enough of them, you are prepared for any situation.

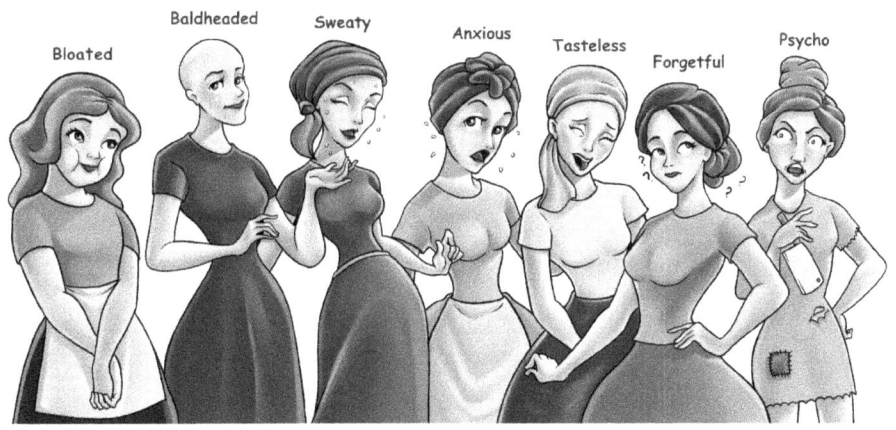

My seven chemo personalities:
Bloated, Baldheaded, Sweaty, Anxious, Tasteless, Forgetful, and Psycho.

Hot flashes, night sweats, mood swings, insomnia, and no taste buds were a few added perks of my cancer destruction process.

Let's start with my mood swings, which varied throughout the day. One minute I was happier than a kid in a toy store; the next, I was a zombie ready to rip someone's face off.

My hot flashes were more like a power surge, an unexpected increase of heat. It felt like my inner child was playing with matches all day long. My best friend became a working fan.

The night sweats were unavoidable, but with my chemo brain, I wasn't sure I was wetting the bed or having night sweats. I was literally a hot mess! A hot mess with no taste.

My tastebuds were long gone. Some days I wasn't sure if I was eating a piece of bread or a piece of metal. It really made no difference; I ate for survival.

Lastly, let me mention my night struggles when the steroids kicked in. I didn't know if I had insomnia or was becoming nocturnal. I counted one sheep, two sheep, a cow, and a pig, Old MacDonald had a farm, hey Macarena! And still, there I was, wide awake. On a lucky day, it would take me three hours, 11 pillow flips, seven different positions, two trips to the bathroom, and a partridge in a pear tree.

These were just a few of the *chemons* and multiple personalities I was fighting. Fun stuff. Did I mention chemo brain? Let me just say it was like having déjà vu and amnesia at the same time. Some days, I felt as if my brain had left. Actually, I still feel that way most days. The point is that all this chemo made my mood not just swing; it bounced, rebounded, fluctuated, and occasionally pirouetted.

No Hair, Who Cares

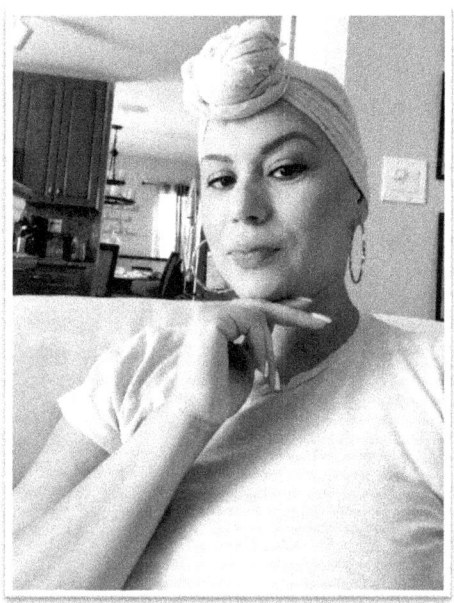

Remember that bomb wig I bought? I was so excited and had been looking forward to wearing it, but it was intolerable. Between the heat and the itchiness, I could not keep it on. Even worse, wearing a wig with no sideburns looked a little weird. It did not look like my hair, at least not to me. So, I wore hats or a scarf most days. This was really a *no hair, who cares* phase. My eyebrows and eyelashes were completely gone, and let me tell you, life is hard without lashes. It's like being double bald.

Bad hair days were a thing of the past, and I couldn't even have bad wig days. Luckily, it was just hair, and it would grow back, I hoped. In the meantime, a pair of big earring hoops with my scarves did wonders. Looking at the bright side, I saved some money on hair products and mascara. At least I had that going for me, which was nice.

Brace Yourself – Weight Gain is Coming

Before cancer, maintaining a healthy weight was a priority for me. I worked out and had a toned physique. I meal-prepped and carefully watched what I ate. Until cancer, when everything went down the drain. Dieting became secondary. Cancer led to chemo, chemo led to weight gain, weight gain led to distress, and distress led me to the fridge. It was challenging to eat healthy when only starchy food had some taste.

I was gaining weight by the minute. Hopping on the scale every week before my infusion was torture. I tried to convince the nurse to skip that part every week. It is said that the number on the scale is just a number, or does that just apply to age? My chemo brain and my body were out of control. The doctor stressed that I needed to be mindful of my weight during treatment, but if he really wanted me to be thin, why would he prescribe me meds that made me fat? I gained 45 lbs. Now that I think about it, I was in shape. Round is a shape! The good thing about being overweight is that it makes it harder to be kidnapped, so I was safe.

I kept reminding myself I was a big cup of wonderful, covered in awesome sauce with a splash of sass and a dash of fat. A few times, I thought of exercising, but chemo had caused me to forget everything; even my muscles had no memory of the weights.

Identity Theft

As my treatment progressed and I transitioned from one chemo to the next, it was evident I was in a fight with cancer. My body was tired and weak from all the cancer destruction happening. The bone pain was insufferable. At times, I thought I would break into pieces. My complexion changed, and my blood cell counts were low, making me look pale and sick. I had not even one follicle of hair left on my body. My nails and tongue were darker than my humor. The ravages of chemo were evident.

By the time I finished my treatment, I was a different person. I was unrecognizable. I had forgotten who I was. The person in the mirror was definitely not me. *It felt like my identity had been stolen.* I went from being a happy, sexy, healthy, and slim woman to a bald, pale, and chunky me. I remember asking for a "smoking hot body" pre-cancer, but somehow there was a mix-up. I had a "smoking body," but due to the hot flashes.

I missed the old me. Tired wasn't a feeling anymore; it was a personality trait. I just wanted to put on an *"Out of Order"* sign and call it a day, all day, every day. Chemo transformed my appearance, which was a tragedy considering I am in the beauty business. I felt like a zombie. I was definitely not a beauty, but I was fighting like a beast.

Blesson: Style begins by looking good, bald, and bare.

Women usually put their self-care and pampering on hold throughout a cancer journey. However, this was not the case for me. Despite my physical changes, I wanted to feel like my fabulous self during this process. So, to ensure I did not neglect myself during this transformation process, I made it a mission to find cancer support groups and activities for women going through cancer. I found a class called "Look Good, Feel Better," which gave cancer patients tips and tricks to look good and fashionable during cancer. Of course, I signed up and sat in the front row.

Beauty has always been my passion, especially since I own a beauty salon. There I was, learning new beauty hacks for my bald self. Style begins by looking good bald and bare. I learned different ways to tie scarves on my head, the best products for my now-sensitive skin, and makeup tips for my nonexistent eyebrows and eyelashes, etc. I have always been able to do my own makeup with ease, but I walked out of there all dolled up with a new perspective of beauty and a bag full of goodies. It was a super fun class. I might not have looked as good as I was used to, but at least I felt good, and that was a win.

Fighting Cancer, Going Through Chemo, and Still Sexy

After attending that class, I felt more motivated to focus on my physical appearance. I became a pro at drawing and shaping my eyebrows. I soon realized that having no eyebrows had its perks; you can draw them depending on your mood.

I also mastered the art of wearing scarves on my head. I had now acquired them in every color for every outfit. Scarves and big hoops were my new fashion statement, and I was rocking it. Of course, there is never a bald moment. The minute I walked into a room with a scarf wrapped around my head, it would alert people that cancer was in the house. Gee, I wonder if this scarf makes me look bald? It felt like a pity stare. Without fail, someone would approach me to ask me or make a comment about my cancer, saying things like, "You don't look sick." Or "You are too young." Or my favorite, "At least you have a nice shaped head" Really? *Yes, cancer has done wonders for my appearance*, I thought. I was *fighting cancer, going through Chemo, and still sexy,* according to others.

I know they were just trying to be nice, and I appreciated it, but the last thing I wanted was to cause pity or have people think I was going to die. So, guess what I did? I pulled out my bomb wig and gave it a second chance. The multiple comments about my bald head were a thing of the past. My wig and I became inseparable. I loved my wig; it went well with my personality and made me look fearless. A good wig can speak louder than words, and my hair would be doing the talking from that point forward. I didn't want to be asked about or talk about cancer; I wanted to be done.

Blesson: When life makes you want to tear your hair out, don't forget you are wearing a wig.

I'm not going to deny that after chemo, I was completely distressed with a capital D, which rhymes with depressed, which stands for stress, and now also possessed, all as a result of the toxins. I felt lost in an emotional nightmare. Chemo had done some serious damage. It is stronger than cancer; like a tsunami, it destroys everything in its path.

The recovery process would require time, patience, and a positive attitude. I wasn't sure how I would rebuild from all the physical and emotional harm. It seemed impossible. I literally wanted to pull my hair out, but I remembered I was wearing a wig.

The point is that I got it done. I fought my chemons, lost my identity, adapted to the new temporary me, and did my best to stay the course. Chemo was tough, but so were my multiple personalities. We all had each other's back. Now I can say, "I'm not Wonder Woman, but I survived chemo, and that's close enough."

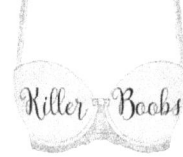

Chapter 10
Cancer Survival Kit

All you need is Love, the cancer card,
uplifting music, and a sense of humor.

CANCER CARD

THIS CARD MAY BE USED TO BE EXCUSED OF ANYTHING

MEMBER SINCE 2018
EXCLUSIVE MEMBERSHIP

There are some things chemo can't avoid;
for everything else, there is the cancer card.

One of the very few advantages of having cancer is that you automatically get instant approval for the very exclusive "Platinum Cancer Card." The card offers incredible benefits like:

1. An elite cancer diagnosis.

2. Unlimited access to the hospital lounge.

3. You can sit back, relax in a comfortable infusion suite and enjoy complimentary cocktails.

4. On-demand access to nurses and doctors.

5. Easy access and unlimited use.

6. It gets you out of social obligations, gatherings, parties, dinners, meetings, and even work at times.

7. Every excuse is valid when you show the card.

This card does wonders, and the perks are endless. I miss that card, probably the only thing I miss from cancer; I wonder if they will ever extend the coverage to survivors?

There is a downside to having this card—the $1600 introductory fee for the diagnosis and the annual membership fee after the treatment can leave you broke. There is always a catch!

Blesson: Music, the original mood-altering, non-fattening wonder drug. Ask your doctor if music is right for you.

Warning: It has been said that exposure to music may cause sudden outbursts of joy, hope, energy, and spontaneous healing. I'm not sure where the warning came from, but I handled it at my own risk.

Music has always been part of my life; it's a way of elevating my moods and reducing stress. In the midst of my chaos, I created a playlist titled *"Songs for a badass on a tough day,"* hoping to feel invincible and hopeful on rough days.

Having this playlist was a form of therapy. Listening to these songs allowed me to visualize my victory and create imaginary music videos with me as the hero of my story. Singing songs like "I Will Survive," "My Fight," and "Titanium" were a few of my go-to songs that I played to help me stay optimistic. These uplifting songs combated the negative committee gatherings in my head, immediately altering my mood and giving me hope. Just in case you are wondering what songs were on my playlist, here are a few:

Badass for Tough Days Playlist

1. I Will Survive – Gloria Gaynor
2. Titanium – David Guetta
3. I Got the Eye of the Tiger – Katy Perry
4. Brave – Sara Bareilles
5. Don't Stop Believing – Journey
6. Hero – Mariah Carey
7. Breakaway – Kelly Clarkson
8. The best day of my life – American Authors
9. Fight Song – Rachel Platten
10. Stand By You – Rachel Platten
11. Rise Up – Andra Day
12. Roar - Katy Perry
13. It's a Beautiful Day – Michael Bublé

14. Ain't No Mountain High Enough – Marvin Gaye

15. I'm Alive – Celine Dion

16. Simply the Best – Tina Turner

17. Dance Again – J. Lo

18. Happy – Pharrell Williams

19. I Believe I Can Fly – R. Kelly

20. Firework – Katy Perry

21. Overcomer – Mandisa

"Resilient people don't take their life too seriously."

Journaling my experiences and making fun of my tragedy through memes and quotes helped me cope while keeping me busy. Inspirational quotes and humor are two traits that identify me and have always been my best form of expression, especially during stressful or traumatic moments. When I find laughter in a difficult situation, it automatically makes me a winner and puts me in control of the outcome. I figured having a positive mental attitude while going through chemo would create more miracles than any drug.

Reading was another powerful tool that helped me throughout. I became a book junkie and read many inspiring stories about cancer survivors who motivated me to continue the fight.

Learning about these women who overcame cancer was encouraging and helped me understand my feelings and emotions. It provided me with a sense of hope, faith, and even laughter, which is exactly the primary purpose of this book.

Identity Under Construction – Please be Patient!

While recovering from the effects of chemo and to avoid falling into a state of depression, I decided to let my creativity flow. I came up with ideas to increase my self-love and self-care. It was essential to handle myself with much love and compassion as I was under construction without an exact completion date.

I got crafty and created a post-chemo care jar and filled it with some of my favorite self-care ideas written on strips of paper. Every day, I would pull out one or two and do the activity selected. This was a daily reminder for me to take care of myself.

Self-Care Jar

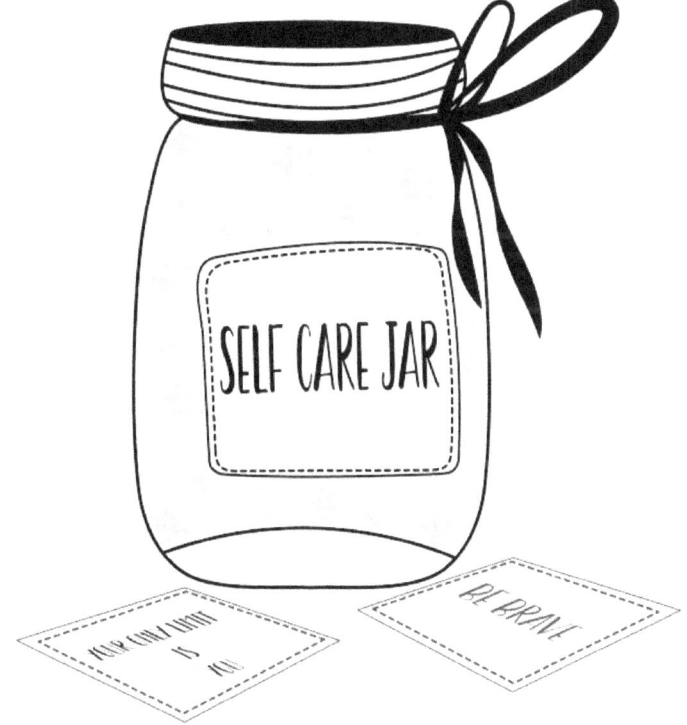

My Jar included the following self-care suggestions:

-Take a few deep Breaths.
-Say a positive Affirmation (see the list attached)
-Say a prayer (see a sample prayer)
-Be grateful for second chances
-Be thankful for my new and improved boobs
-Read something inspirational
-Listen to a bad-ass song
-Go for a walk
-Do some stretches
-Dress up and feel pretty
-Take a cute selfie
-Call a friend
-Sleep in
-Post a funny meme about my current situation
-Put on my bomb wig and some make up and go for a ride with my kids
-Watch a funny movie
-Write in my journal
-Read a few chapters of my favorite book
-Eat my favorite meal
-Dance to my favorite music
-Play a board game with my kids.
-Go out for a long early-morning walk
-Watch Netflix with the family
-Take a long bath.
-Create a collage of the future new and improved me

The Cancerenity Prayer

God Grant me the sanity to accept that I have killer boobs,
The courage to endure the endless side effects of my treatment.
And just enough chemo to give me superpowers.

Amen.

Affirmations

- *Cancer chose the wrong girl.*
- *I am a slaying warrior ninja fighting Goddess.*
- *My God is stronger than my breast cancer.*
- *I am a badass mom beating cancer.*
- *I have 99 problems, but a bad boob ain't one;-)*
- *I will beat cancer one cocktail at a time.*
- *I must continue my quest to slay my tumor with sass and humor.*
- *I will keep going forward even if my hair falls out.*
- *I am a big cup of wonderful, covered in awesome sauce with a splash of chemo and superpowers.*
- *My boobs have gone through thick and thin, but life is too precious to let cancer win.*
- *I am HEALarious.*
- *I beat cancer; there is no stopping me now.*

Blesson: Think positive! For example, "My boobs tried to kill me, and I thought, Wow I'm glad I killed them first."

Life doesn't always go the way we expect it to, but when things go wrong, we must take a moment to be positive and thankful for the many other things that are going right. Having a positive attitude, keeping my sunny side up, and practicing self-care did not mean I was ignoring the negative; it meant I could overcome it.

I had many difficult days where faith, hope, and positivity were not clear, but when those days came, I had my toolbox of essentials to find comfort and keep me going.

I truly believe that my ability to find positivity, humor, and irony in this challenging situation made me resilient.

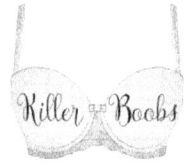

Chapter 11

I Don't Mean to Brag But... I Just Beat Cancer

Gone But Not Forgotten

I have exited Cancerville. Now what???

There is no question that beating cancer was one of my greatest accomplishments.

I should've been ecstatic and relieved, but I was uncertain. I felt more lost than a chameleon in a bag of skittles. When I started my treatment, my goal was to finish, but I didn't really know what to do once I finished. I went from having all the attention from family and friends to having very minimal attention. I was fine now, according to others. Where did everybody go?

My doctor visits were less frequent, and my friends and family slowly returned to their normal lives. *Hello!! I'm here! Don't forget me.* The negative committee in my head trying to get attention reminded me. *I'm still emotional.* I was healed from cancer, but now I had an emotional overflow; not sure if I felt invincible or just emotionally numb. I wish I could have told Alexa to turn off my emotions, but she wasn't around. My identity was still nowhere to be found. That was a good thing because if I did not know who I was, then cancer won't find me again. Right? The fear of recurrence was inevitable, and it lingers in my mind. Technically, I am not a survivor until I hit the five-year mark. One more year and it will be official.

Hey Google, is My Cancer Back?

Have you heard of Dr. Google? Well, that is the doctor you go to when you have a headache to find out if it is a brain tumor. The first couple of visits to my oncologist were filled with anxiety, and I wasn't sure if I was in danger or just being paranoid. Doctor, everything hurts, and I have a paper cut. Am I going to die? Not everything is cancer, he often reminds me. Don't worry; you are not going to die. Well, yes, you are going to die eventually but not right now. Gee, Doc! Thanks a lot!

Post-chemo, a PET scan was ordered to ensure there were no signs of cancer in my body. One more PET scan, and I'll glow in the dark! Bring it on. *I have the results of your PET and CT scans*, the doctor called to inform me. My heart dropped; the scanxiety was real. You're safe; no evidence of cancer, *but…* you are officially a hypochondriac. Oh my, is that going to kill me?

Just Because I Look OK Does Not Mean I am

My role as Super Woman and a cool mom beating cancer remained, but on the inside, I was still fighting my demons. Fear, readjusting, and accepting my new reality was tough. I felt like a long-time prisoner being released from jail and learning to readjust to society. What will my new post-cancer life be like? What changes do I need to make? How do I deal with my new body? What am I going to eat for dinner? Profound thoughts, especially this last one. This is when the negative committee had some serious gatherings in my head. I needed emotional support more than ever. Some days all I needed was laughter, but on others, I needed strength and to let out a good cry. I did have a dog, but after hearing me whine on those sad days, I could tell that being an emotional support dog was not his thing. I could tell by his look what he was thinking. "Deal with it. You just beat cancer; you're Wonder Woman."

Installing Boobs, Please Wait!

The minute my treatment was over, I immediately requested the doctor remove the chemo port. They usually recommend keeping it there for a few months post-chemo just in case, but I was done with cancer. I wanted it out and was ready to start my new life and get my new boobs.

One thing I looked forward to the most after finishing my treatment was removing those hard rocks off my chest and having normal implants. It was a way of getting back to some kind of normality.

The day has come. My boobs were going to be installed at last. The moment I had been waiting for, even before cancer—small, perky new pair of boobs. I was so excited. "Please, Doc, I don't want big boobs!" I exclaimed right before surgery. "No worries," he said, and off I went. The good news is that the reconstruction surgery went well. My new boobs were now installed. The bad news was they were definitely a tenacious DD. Now I really did not know who I was with these two new knockers.

At first, the doctor said not to worry; they were just swollen and within a few months, the swelling would go down. I waited, and waited and waited for almost a year and the knockers were still hard and intact. Now what? My only chance to get small boobs was ruined. This cannot be happening to me. I had worse luck than a bald guy who just won a comb.

Killer Boob to the Rescue

Remember my infamous killer boob? She was back. She wanted to make her presence known. She was not happy, and neither was I. She was rejecting the implant. Of course, she was; she's always been a rebel. For the first time in a long time, we agreed. I did not approve of the size and did not feel comfortable. I was very self-conscious when going into a room because it was as if my boobs were yelling, "Hello, here we are. Take a look!"

The boob continued to bother me like crazy. The implant was not a good fit (or a good size). The discomfort was perpetual, and I could not bear the pain. I needed to change the implants, or they would kill me. I can't deny it, I was secretly happy because this was my chance to get smaller boobs finally. Off to a third breast surgery I went. Goodbye boobs!

Fifty Shades of Grey

My hair started growing back right before chemo ended. Ugh! Now I had to start shaving my armpits again. My short gray hair was out. Yes, gray hair. I said it. Or should I just call it stress highlights? Whatever, at least it was growing back. It was like the fifty shades of grey on my head. My short hair looked like I had received a botched haircut from my worst enemy—no shape or style. I was still filled with toxins, so I refused to use hair dye to let my body rest from any other chemicals. This is when I really took advantage of my wigs. By this point, I had acquired a few different ones, even a hat with a ponytail, you know, to wear to the gym. I had to cover all my bases. I'm a planner like that, but you probably know that by now.

I didn't want my wig to fall off when I was working out at the gym. Can you imagine that scene? It would have led to canceling my membership. How tragic!

Short Hair, Who Cares?

After a year, my hair had grown to a decent short length, so I decided it was time to style it. I wasn't sure if I was going to rock it as I had never had short hair before, but again, I thought it was the perfect opportunity to try a different look, let my hair do the talking, and see how it felt. I went to the salon to have it colored, shaped, and styled into a nice, trendy pixie cut. I finally did it. It was quite liberating, and I felt free. I left with a *short hair, don't care* attitude. They say there is something about women with short hair that screams power, so there I was, a super powerful survivor. I got many compliments, but I wasn't comfortable yet, so I kept alternating between my short hair and my bomb wigs, depending on my mood. It was quite fun. Wigs can be addictive; I can certainly understand why Beyoncé wears them.

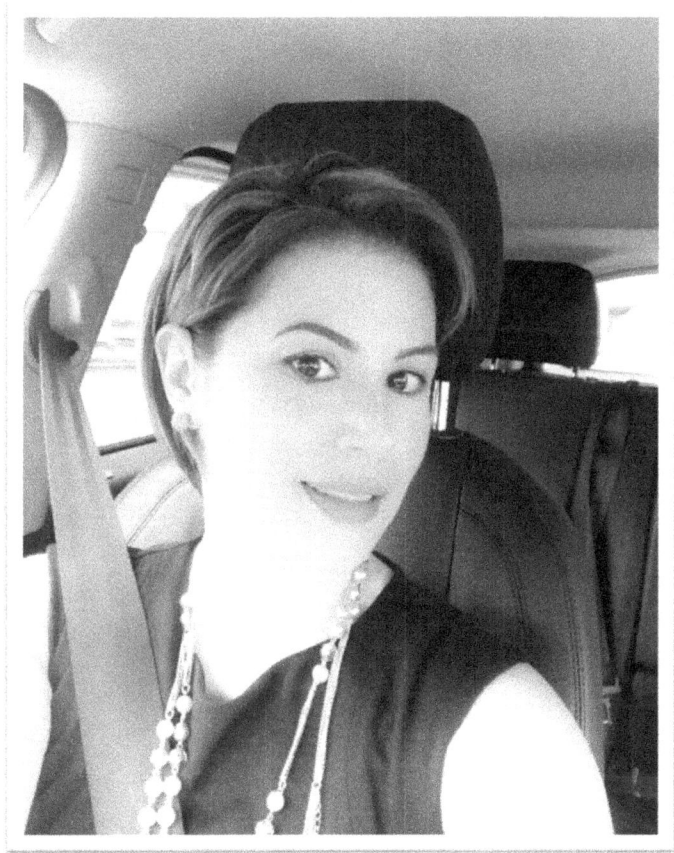

I Came Out With Short Hair.

Blesson: Shaken, Not Stirred

Exiting Cancerville was tough. It was the beginning of a new life filled with uncertainty and unpredictability. Loneliness and fear were two emotions I couldn't control. I had to learn to take a breather and regain my strength. I got knocked down but realized I needed to get up and find ways to reinvent and reincorporate myself into my new normal.

I did not allow my emotions to distract me from what needed to be done. I focused on my healing and on accepting my new reality. I learned to stay informed about the things I must do as a survivor and stay healthy. I was certainly shaken but not stirred, and life needed to go on. I was not meant to die at 39; I had unfinished business, and I needed to pick up right where I left off before Cancer.

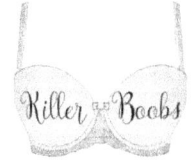

Chapter 12

Until Cancer Do Us Part

Couples that hustle together, don't always stay together.

The day we got married, my husband and I promised to be together in good and bad, sickness and health, but not until cancer did us part. This was definitely not in our happy family life plan. While I can't blame cancer for our marriage failing, it certainly came at a time when our marriage was debilitating. Without going into too many details about it (let's not lose focus here. This is a book about cancer, not about my love life), I would like to share some of the history of our love story.

We married in 2004 in New York. Like most young couples, we had many dreams and aspirations for our future. Fourteen years later, we moved to Florida, bought a business, and had two beautiful and healthy children. He and I were always a great team. Our roles were well established: he was the go-getter and opportunity seeker, and I was the supporter who made things happen. Like vitamins, we supplemented each other's daily minimum requirements.

After going into business together, our roles reversed. I became the decision-maker, and he took on more of a support role. It didn't really matter because we had big plans, and our focus was to succeed. For many years, we worked ceaselessly. Perhaps working long hours and being so focused on success caused our relationship to suffer. Running a business with your spouse can be tricky since different personalities and mindsets often lead to the wrong outcome, making it difficult to set personal and professional boundaries. We faced many difficulties and had to jump many hurdles, but we always managed to fight for our marriage and continue building our empire.

In Sickness and in Health

When cancer paid us an unexpected visit, my husband kept his promise made in our vows; he stood by me, solid as a rock. It's funny, though, because I would often complain about his lack of romanticism, but he proved me wrong with his acts of kindness. He shaved my head, changed my bloody drains, made my green smoothies, carried me to and from bed, dealt with my multiple chemons, and accepted having a breastless wife. If this isn't romance, then what is?

He truly was there for me in sickness, probably much more than in health. He had to cope with his wife battling cancer, fulfill his role as a father, and take full charge of our business. Not everyone is equipped to handle all these changes at once.

People always tend to care for the person going through cancer, but not many consider the needs of the patient's spouse. The lack of support and empathy for caregivers and their suffering and fear is greater than we might think. My husband always tried to act as if everything would be OK, but I'm sure he was hurting and fearful of what might happen. Despite this, he was strong and stayed the course. However, by the end of my treatment, he was obviously worn out and overwhelmed from all the added obligations.

Marriages are Made in Heaven. But so are Thunder, Lightning, Tornadoes, and Hail.

Our relationship went from love and happiness to doubts, fights, stress, pain, and finally, regret. Our conversations became shorter and less meaningful. We became two strangers living together in the same house. Our silence meant we were tired of fighting and didn't have the energy to argue. Well, at least I didn't because I was under the influence of chemo, with my multiple personalities.

This new dynamic created complex emotions that strained our marriage. The constant disagreements, my multiple personalities, the stress of the salon, the cancer, the lightning, the tornados, the hail, the dog, the cat. Oh no, we didn't have a cat. I get carried away listing the many reasons for our failed marriage. Whatever the cause, it was evident that our love had faded.

I Loved You with All my Boobs, but They are Now Gone

My children and my spouse were my motivation to keep going through cancer.

Family is one of the most important values to me. I thought my family life would go back to normal after I was done with cancer. I was ready to take my life back and appreciate the second chance to live and have a loving family. I wanted to start from scratch and do all the things that we hadn't previously done as a family because of work and other distractions. I wanted to be the perfect mom and wife this time around. I had it all mapped out: have fun, enjoy each other, travel and create memories, and be present. But I could not have been further from reality. It was over, just like my boobs, and we could not repair the damage. I was not ready for another unexpected plot twist. The timing was terrible; I had already lost too many things too soon: my identity, my boobs, and now my marriage.

The Inspirational Mantra

"Never get used to what doesn't make you happy." I will never forget that mantra because it was the screensaver on my husband's cell phone. I am not judging him; I am sure he had his reasons, but it was a clear message to me that I was not part of his happiness. It was a hard pill to swallow, but I was a pro at taking all sorts of pills at this point, so what's one more? Unfortunately, this one almost made me choke. This truly was one of the darkest moments of my life. My heart had been ripped into a million pieces. I felt lost and cried for weeks. Deep inside, I knew it was over, and I should let go. The love was gone, but I did not want to give up. I wanted to fight for this as hard as I fought cancer.

Where is the Parenting Manual?

Although we never argued in front of our children and tried to be as civil as possible, I am sure they noticed the coldness between us long before we split. Children are very intuitive; they often know more than what we give them credit for. I felt bad for them. Right after witnessing their mother battle cancer, they now had to endure their parents separating. This was going to disrupt their lives. My heart was heavy. As a mother, I was worried about their mental well-being because so many changes were happening simultaneously. How can I help them avoid the pain? Why isn't there a parenting manual to deal with these situations? Why hasn't someone come up with one yet? I really could have used it then, and even now, actually! Anyhow, we did our best to handle it, given the circumstances. I knew it was the best choice for us because we were unhappy, and unhappy parents led to unhappy kids. Our precious children deserved to have happy parents so they wouldn't end up emotionally damaged or grow up with the wrong concept of love.

Blesson: When someone walks away from you, it's not the end of your story. It's the end of their life in your story.

Our breakup was unexpected and heartbreaking, but we clearly failed to ensure each other's needs were met. We both expected too much and didn't deliver. We failed in so many ways except in conceiving two beautiful children. We were not meant to end up together despite all our efforts. However, there is always a *blesson* to be learned.

First, one should always have the courage to walk away from what doesn't make us happy and not settle, as my husband's mantra stated.

Second, as difficult as it might seem during that loss, life does go on and will eventually reward you with a new hello. If cancer didn't kill me, a divorce wouldn't either.

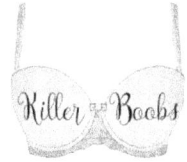

Chapter 13
A Little Stitious

I am purposefully skipping this chapter.

It's not that I am SUPERstitious, but I am a little stitious. I already had killer boobs, so I'm not taking any chances.

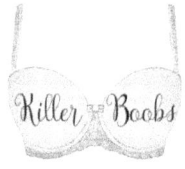

Chapter 14

Well, That Didn't Go As Planned!

Have you ever sat down and thought...
Damn, I've been through a lot of S#!t!

This chapter title sums up my year in one sentence. A lot has happened!

I had killer boobs, got a double mastectomy, went through chemo, had six surgeries, a loss of identity, a failed marriage, and became a newly-single mother. This was indeed my year! Boy, I've been through a lot of s#!t. I wonder if it was because I didn't forward that email to ten people?

At this point in my life, I was more baffled than Chris Rock at the Oscars when Will Smith smacked him across the face. I know God wouldn't give me anything I couldn't handle, but I wished he didn't trust me so much. I really needed someone to hug me and say, "I know life is hard, you are going to be ok; here is a chocolate and $6 million." OK, maybe not the hug or the chocolate, but at least the $6 million? Was that too much to ask for? C'mon, please! I didn't understand how my perfectly imperfect life could change so much in such a short time. My life was like a test I didn't study for. Where do I go from here? I really needed help—professional help… A stylist, chef, maid, and personal trainer. You know, help with basic things like that would have done it, at least until I found myself. I needed to adapt to my new life and my boobs.

My path was not clear, and I was scared. I was in a mental war. The negative committee in my head was constantly trying to show up, and some days, it even took over, but enough was enough! It was pep talk time. Hello. You are a badass mom who fought cancer like a *tumornator*. You have great new boobs! You got this, and you're fabulous. Love you!

She Remembered Who She Was, and the Game Changed

The pity party was over, and it was time to get my life back. I was the only person responsible for saving myself and figuring things out. Where do I start? How do I rebuild the broken pieces of who I was? For starters, I did not like my image, except for my boobs—those were perfect, but I was uncomfortable with my body. Here we go again. Stop it; you already know what happened the last time you were unhappy with a part of your body!

Let's face it. After going through two life-altering circumstances—cancer and a separation—and being bald and overweight, building my confidence was definitely something I needed to work on. I felt unattractive and needed to lose the extra weight I had borrowed to protect my body from chemo (I always blame it on chemo). It was time to get back to the gym and get my sexy back. Looking at the bright side, the breakup did accelerate the weight loss a bit. At least I had that! I put together an action plan and started working on my mindset, self-development, and spirituality. I also created a workout routine and a meal plan and decided to get to work.

I was very disciplined and committed to achieving my inner and outer transformation. In a few weeks, I started feeling better physically and emotionally. I noticed my body was looking toned, and my self-esteem started improving. My hair was growing back, and the new and improved version of me was finally starting to blossom. I felt comfortable and happy, and things began to fall into place. My daily routines, my life as a newly single mother, and my social life all started to feel normal. I was rediscovering and reinventing myself, and it felt good—great, actually. I had forgotten who I was for a long time, doing things out of habit and in autopilot mode. I was a bit lost, but It was OK because I was back and the game had changed.

> **Blesson: Don't just survive; that's not what you were made for. Instead, live with purpose and passion.**

If Not Now, When?

During that time of self-discovery and self-reflection, I really looked inward and asked myself hard questions about my life's happiness and purpose. I realized that I was a missing piece to my professional puzzle—there was a lack of fulfillment. I was not living with purpose and had been ignoring my potential. Yes, I had a thriving business that brought me joy, but I had forgotten my passion, teaching and mentoring. That always brought me so much happiness and satisfaction, and I needed to reconnect with it. I had gotten a little sidetracked with the business, kids, and life, but it was time to refocus and go back to doing what I was born to do.

I decided to go back to school and further my education as a coach and obtained a life coaching certification. If not now, when? My calling has always been to impact lives and serves others through teaching, mentoring, and leadership. As of today, I have helped hundreds of people through seminars, classes, and one-on-one coaching. I even created my coaching methodology, Valor-Arte—the art of valuing yourself to empower *women to embrace their self-worth, regain their confidence, and become the best version of themselves,* just as I did. Perhaps I needed cancer to shake me a little to wake me up to reconnect and find myself.

"Hard times are like a washing machine, they twist, turn, and knock us around, but in the end, we come out cleaner, brighter, and better than before."

Working on myself inside and out after everything I had endured was one of my greatest accomplishments. It definitely helped boost my self-confidence and self-esteem. After such a transformation, great opportunities came my way. I don't mean to brag, but let me tell you that life after cancer has gotten really fun. For starters, I made it to the top ten at *HERS Fitness* magazine, thanks to my toned physique. I also have been invited as a keynote speaker to several Cancer fundraiser events and radio shows. More recently, I participated in three bathing suit fashion runways. Lastly, I received the "Women of Power Award 2022." And to top it all off, I became a published author. As J. Lo would say, "I'm just getting started."

Blesson: I survived what I thought would kill me. Now it's time to straighten my crown and move forward like the queen that I am.

Perhaps I did not deserve all that happened to me. Maybe I did, but regardless, I admired my strength, bravery, and resilience in overcoming the darkest moments of my life. Cancer is an ugly word with a scary meaning. Instead of defining me, it built up my character and shaped me into the woman I am today. It wasn't fun. I had good days, bad days, fun days, overwhelming days, exhausting days, I am going to die days, I'm Superwoman days, and I can't go on days, but I still showed up like the fighter that I am every day.

Overcoming cancer revealed beautiful gifts: courage, faith, and hope. It made me want to live with intention—bolder and bigger. It forced me to take life less seriously and appreciate and savor every moment. I certainly learned the meaning of resilience. That year, I met the most broken version of myself and the strongest. After standing up to cancer, nothing else that comes my way seems too difficult. Today, as I count my blessings, I feel healthier, stronger, and more active than ever. I can confidently say that I survived what I thought would kill me. Now it's time to straighten my crown and move forward like the queen that I am.

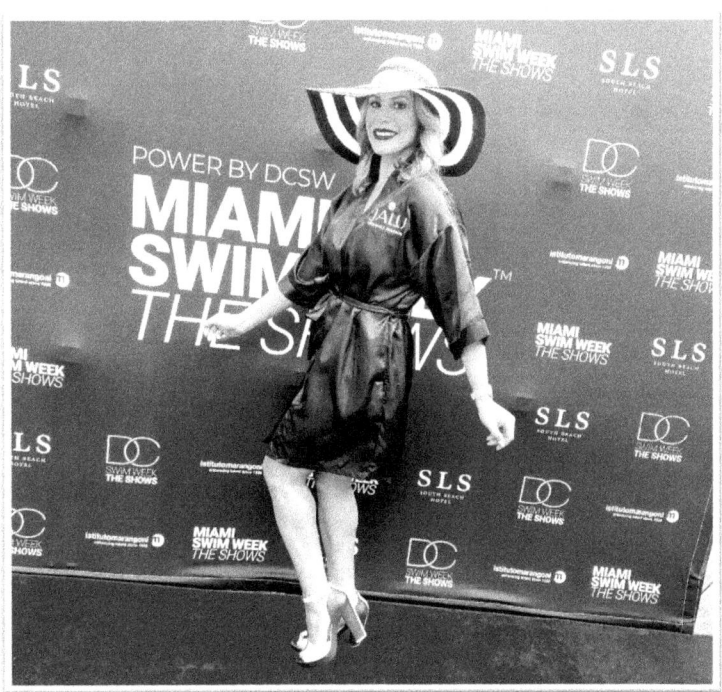

Note to self:

**On a particularly rough day when I think I can't possibly endure;
I remind myself that my track record for getting
through bad days so far has been 100%.**

And that is pretty awesome!

—Aga's Book of Miracles

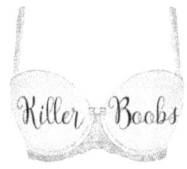

Chapter 15

Wait, One More Thing...

Why do good people get cancer?

After writing the last chapter of this book and sending it to my editor, a very good friend called asking me for some advice. Someone close to her had recently been diagnosed with breast cancer, and she wanted to know what helped me during my journey and what encouraging gifts might help her friend. I recommended some books that I had read that helped me. Then I thought, "OMG, my book would have been perfect for her!" Unfortunately, it hadn't been published yet, and cancer doesn't wait. What a bummer!

We continued to talk about the C-word and questioned, "Why do good people get cancer?" Right then, I realized, "Holy crap, I forgot to include that in my book. How could I?" Well, it's the chemo brain still acting up; it lasts for years. The point is that this is a common question many people ask when cancer hits home and one that I am still trying to answer. Was it because I didn't go to church on Sundays or because when I was six, I lied to my mom about eating all my food when I was really throwing it out the window? Oh no, it was because I failed to feed the parrots when my mom left me in charge, and they died. Damn karma! For sure, this had to be the consequence of one or all my past sins. I did a lot of blaming and questioning. I even had the audacity to question God, as if He had anything to do with it. I mean, I was the one who forgot to feed the birds.

Time to Freak Out... Panic First, Think Later

When I was first diagnosed, I became so paranoid about anything going in or on my body that I stopped eating. Food causes cancer! I quit using lotions, soaps, perfumes, detergents, and even deodorants—not such a good idea. Who said deodorant is optional? After doing thorough research on Google, it was obvious that my cancer resulted from food and harsh chemicals. I completely switched all my products to non-GMO, paraben-free, oil-free, gluten-free, sugar-free, fat-free, air-free, etc. Basically, I only drank water from Whole Foods.

After consulting with my oncologist about all the changes I had made voluntarily, he suggested trying to live as normal a life as possible since nothing has been proven 100% to cause cancer. My research continued, and I met with a nutritionist to completely adjust my diet. I was sure something specific must have caused it, and I needed to know what it was. Perhaps it was the chocolate chip cookies I ate the week before. Funny enough, little needed to change as I had already been on a healthy journey. So what was it then? I had no choice but to do some serious introspection and draw the best conclusions I could on my own.

Buildup of Emotions with a High Dose of Stress

Although there is no scientific evidence of what causes cancer, I attribute my cancer to a buildup of repressed emotions with a high dose of stress.

As I shared with you in earlier chapters, I was the true definition of a perfectionist. In my life, everything had to be flawless according to my standards. Anyone who knows me can attest to that. While many people will take pride in believing this is a great quality to have, that is far from the truth.

Perfectionism can be a double-edged sword—it can be a strength and a weakness. It's not economical, and the price I was paying for it was pretty high. I put unnecessary pressure on myself, often leading to frustration and burnout. My perfectionism was a representation of my wanting to have control over everything. It's not like I was a control freak; I just liked to have things my way.

Forgive and Forget? I'm Neither Jesus nor do I Have Alzheimer's

As much as I wanted to say that I had no resentment stored in my heart, the truth is that over the years, I had been stacking a mixture of disappointments, bitterness, and emotional traumas. Unfortunately, I am the type to bottle things up inside and not express emotions. In retrospect, I realized that I had suppressed many negative feelings. I had a lack of forgiveness that was holding me hostage. Many situations that occurred in my personal and professional life had me angry—too many setbacks, betrayals, backstabbing, etc. How can I forgive and forget? I'm neither Jesus nor do I have Alzheimer's, is what I usually thought to myself. However, I am sure all of these toxic emotions contributed to my cancer illness. As the saying goes, "If you are not speaking it, you are storing it, and that is heavy."

Blesson: The mind and body are not separate. What affects one affects the other.

While I was great at caring for my body, my mind was not at ease. My daily obligations and responsibilities were having an adverse reaction to my mental health. I even forgot how to laugh and have fun. When you are not at peace with your mind, your body starts deteriorating, and no workout can offset that mental war. This was happening to me. I was so stressed out that I felt as if I did not have control over my body, and nothing made sense. I constantly felt sick and tired.

Now I understand why I was constantly exhausted; I was fighting a mental war every day. It was hard for me to admit my emotions. I have worked on my personal development for many years, and I felt ashamed to think something could be wrong with me. After my treatment, I decided to get a life coach as part of my healing. Throughout the sessions, I confronted my emotions and freed myself from my mental war to move on. I decided to make healthy choices for my body AND my mind.

Admitting our emotions and feelings makes us vulnerable, which is hard, but as Brenè Brown says, "Vulnerability is not weakness; it's our most accurate measure of courage." It is OK not to be OK. But it is not OK to live in denial. Only when I started being honest with myself and recognizing my pain, anger, and shortcomings was I able to heal. In fact, I became mentally *healarious*.

Blesson: You have been assigned this mountain to show others that it can be moved.

So, why does cancer happen to good people like me? After much thought, I determined it happens for many reasons:

1. To teach lessons, or as I call them, *Blessons*, so we can make necessary adjustments in our lives. I clearly needed to stop controlling everything, learn to relax, let go, and have faith that things would work out.

2. Why not me? Obviously, I can handle it. God trusts me. He knows I am a badass. Besides, who else would I have preferred to get cancer? Let's just say I took one for the team.

3. God wanted to remind me that I was made for greatness. He had to shake me a little to test my strength and ignite the fire within me to live to my full potential.

Final Message

Cancer will change your life, and the change can be beautiful.
—Jane Cook

There is life after chemo, surgeries, divorce, or any other traumatic experience that we may encounter. Things will pass. We must have faith, stay strong, be awesome, and most importantly, learn our *blessons*.

Below are some important *Cancer Blessons* to remember:

1. All lumps are not equal. One must learn the difference.

2. When diagnosed with Cancer, you have only two choices:

    You CANsurvive or you CANsurrender.

3. When life doesn't go as planned, yell "Plot twist!" and move on.

4. Breasts are just lumps of fat that make us look sexy. Sometimes we don't need the extra fat.

5. When your boobs try to kill you, kill them first and get new ones.

6. If you put on a little weight while going through chemo, remember that fat people are harder to kidnap.

7. Losing your hair during chemo ensures you won't have bad hair days and saves you tons of money on hair products.

8. When your hair falls off, get a bomb wig and move on.

9. Hair, no hair, some hair or wig, you are still you, and you are beautiful.

10. You can fight cancer, go through chemo, and still look sexy.

11. Resilient people don't take life too seriously.

12. Always keep calm but check your boobs; you already know mine tried to kill me.

13. Remember to touch your bumps for any lumps because mammogramming your boobs is better than Instagramming them.

14. When you are going through a hard time and wonder where God is, remember that the teacher is always quiet during the test.

15. When everything else fails, family is always there, like a good support bra.

16. You can't die if you have unfinished business, be a shark and attack cancer.

17. When the negative committee wants to meet inside your head, tell it to sit down and shut up; you are in control.

18. Attitude is everything, so pick a good one. A positive mindset and lots of laughter are always the perfect prescriptions.

19. Surviving doesn't just mean staying alive; it means you will find your passion and live with purpose. It's time to shine bright like a diamond.

And lastly...

20. If you have a tumor and it's loaded with cancer, suck it out, slice it up, and nuke it. Then say… "Take that, Cancer!"

Congratulations....

You are now a certified badass in the fight against cancer!

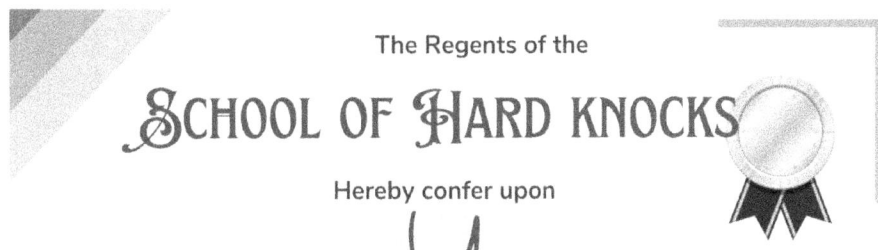

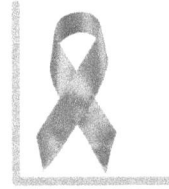

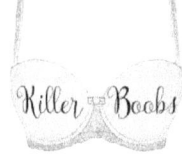

About the Author

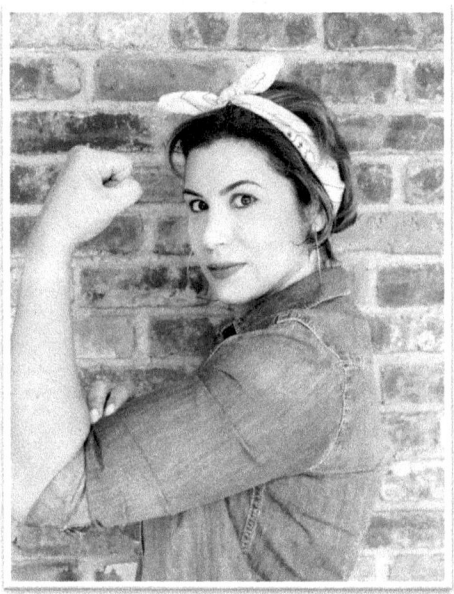

Lucy Beato is a multi-faceted businesswoman, educator, life coach, and author who expertly balances business, career, and family as a single mother.

Like most women, Lucy dreamed of a stable life filled with love, laughter, and fulfillment. Her dreams changed dramatically when she was diagnosed with breast cancer at thirty-nine, followed by a failed marriage. Where circumstances like these defeat many women, and while she didn't know it then, these tragedies affirmed her calling and ultimate purpose to commit to cracking the code and discovering the skills used by those who overcome adversity and succeed. She set out on this quest and was determined to bring back the tools to teach others how it can be done and to give them the opportunities to find hope, strength, and humor where it seems there is none. After spending years unlocking these secrets and crafting a results-driven curriculum, she offers practical guidance and solutions today to women all over the world with her coaching methodology.

www.ingramcontent.com/pod-product-compliance
Lightning Source LLC
LaVergne TN
LVHW051842080426
835512LV00018B/3024